the feel-good
FAMILY FOOD PLAN

EVERYTHING YOU NEED TO FEED YOUR FAMILY WELL, EVERY DAY

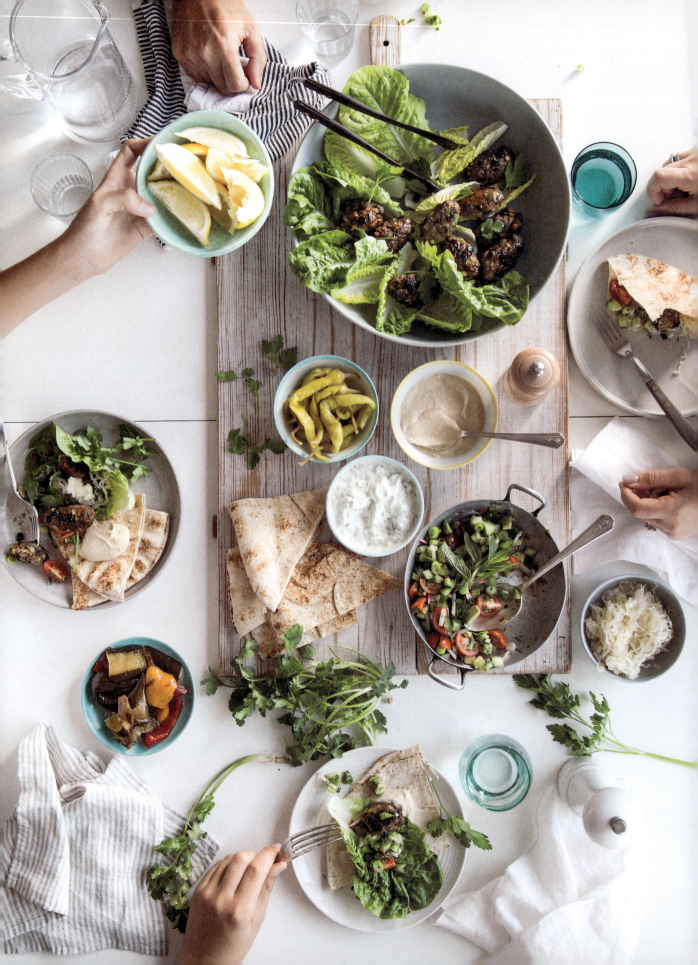

Australia's most trusted nutritionist **Dr JOANNA McMILLAN**

with Melissa Clark

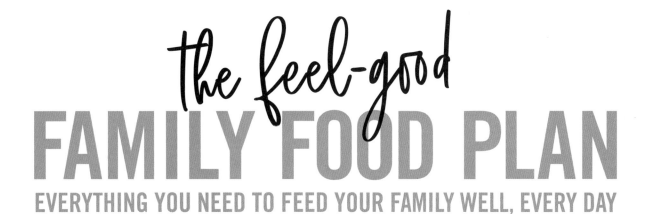

the feel-good FAMILY FOOD PLAN

EVERYTHING YOU NEED TO FEED YOUR FAMILY WELL, EVERY DAY

murdoch books

Sydney | London

CONTENTS

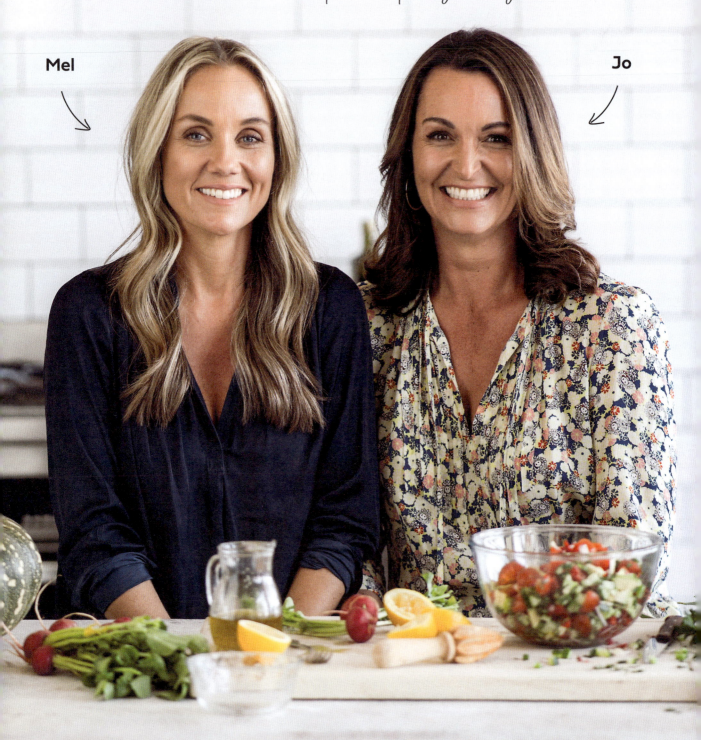

Our goal is for you to feel confident that you can feed your family delicious, nutritious meals... and for food to be a pleasurable part of your family life.

Mel

Jo

WHAT IS A HEALTHY DIET?

WHY THE CONFUSION?

The purpose of this book is to give you the confidence to know that you are feeding your family as best you can, the tools to help you deal with the many difficult food situations that can arise, the tricks to making mealtimes easier and within budget while minimising food waste, and the inspiration to make food a pleasurable and delicious part of your family life.

Before we look at what constitutes a healthy diet, let's first address why there is so much confusion over defining healthy eating by looking at the example of eggs. As I was writing this book, I was contacted by a journalist about a study that had just been published, which called back into question the healthfulness of eggs.

Eggs were 'out' in the days of low-cholesterol eating, back in the 1970s and early '80s, only to be later exonerated as newer research showed that dietary cholesterol really didn't have too much effect on blood cholesterol. Then, as low-carb diets rotated back into fashion (that's right, they're not new!), eggs were all the rage for breakfast. And now a new study has come along that claims that the more eggs people eat, the higher their risk of heart disease!

If you are one of those to throw up your hands in frustration and feel even more confused as to what to feed your family, let me reassure you of this fact: *we really do understand how to best feed the human race. It's not all that complicated, although it can be hard to execute for all sorts of reasons.* Nutrition research might still be debating and studying the nuances and finer details, but the big picture is clear. Don't allow sensationalist media headlines to distract you from this fact.

THE FOUNDATIONS OF A HEALTHY DIET

Back to eggs. If you love them, rest assured that we use them frequently in this book. Eggs are a whole food, delivering an impressive array of nutrients, and so I continue to count them as a wonderfully nutritious food for your family.

The different research results highlight just how tricky studying diet can be. Think of the different ways you could eat eggs. Do you eat them fried in refined seed oil, a potential source of harmful trans fats? Do you eat them with bacon, sausages or other processed meats? As part of a big breakfast with hash browns and buttered white bread? Scrambled with loads of cream? Or do you poach or boil them and have them with avocado toast, or as an omelette with spinach, mushrooms and other vegies? You can see that these different ways of eating eggs have different potentials to impact health. This makes it really, really hard to look at that food in isolation.

Ultimately, what is important is your dietary pattern or the way you put foods together – the overall variety of foods that you consume from week to week, and the balance of different foods that ensure you get all of the nutrients you need.

Recognise that there are many ways to put together a healthy diet. What works for one person might not be right for another, but we do all share the same foundations. So choose a diet of whole foods, including plentiful plants (whether or not you choose to also consume animal foods), with minimal (or no) ultra-processed food.

Your dietary pattern is what determines the overall quality of your diet.

A TEMPLATE FOR HEALTHY EATING

I developed the Dr Joanna Plate over years of working with clients to help them build a visual image of how to balance different foods at each meal. In essence, the Plate is your foundation to start building a healthy diet for your own family. Pictured opposite are four versions of the Plate. For adults, aim for half of the plate to be vegies, a quarter of the plate a protein-rich food and a quarter of the plate a smart carb, and then add a healthy fat (e.g. use extra virgin olive oil for cooking). For teens and younger kids who need a more energy-dense meal, the division is a third for each category, again with a healthy fat-rich food added.

The Plate isn't set in stone because flexibility is key. Everyone's dietary needs are different – sometimes very different. Little kids have smaller tummies and need to eat more energy-dense meals and, since they can't eat as much in one go, they also need to eat more often. Very active teenagers with a heavy sports load need a bigger Plate for starters, but they will also need more smart carbs to fuel their activity. A sedentary dad or mum who spends much of their day at a desk doesn't need such a high level of carbohydrate for fuel and is much more likely to need to control their energy intake to maintain a healthy weight. For them, loading the Plate with vegies will help keep the kilojoules down, while keeping up the nutrients and volume of food.

The beauty of the Plate is that you can use it to put together a meal at home or to choose from a restaurant or takeaway menu. That's important because, although I encourage families to prepare most meals at home, most of us eat out more than generations past. And let's be perfectly honest, there will be nights when takeaway is the preferable option, no matter how inspiring we manage to make our recipes! You can still choose healthier options in these situations and you can almost always make the Plate work with a little know-how. It might be as simple as skipping the fries and adding a side of steamed or stir-fried vegies, or choosing brown rice over white and adding a salad.

THE DR JOANNA PLATE

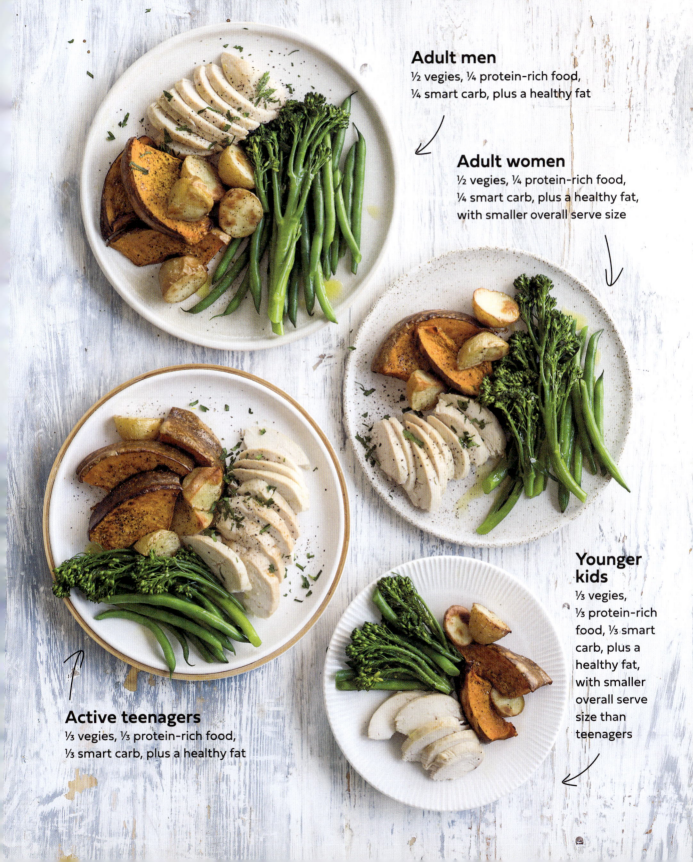

Adult men
½ vegies, ¼ protein-rich food,
¼ smart carb, plus a healthy fat

Adult women
½ vegies, ¼ protein-rich food,
¼ smart carb, plus a healthy fat,
with smaller overall serve size

Younger kids
⅓ vegies,
⅓ protein-rich
food, ⅓ smart
carb, plus a
healthy fat,
with smaller
overall serve
size than
teenagers

Active teenagers
⅓ vegies, ⅓ protein-rich food,
⅓ smart carb, plus a healthy fat

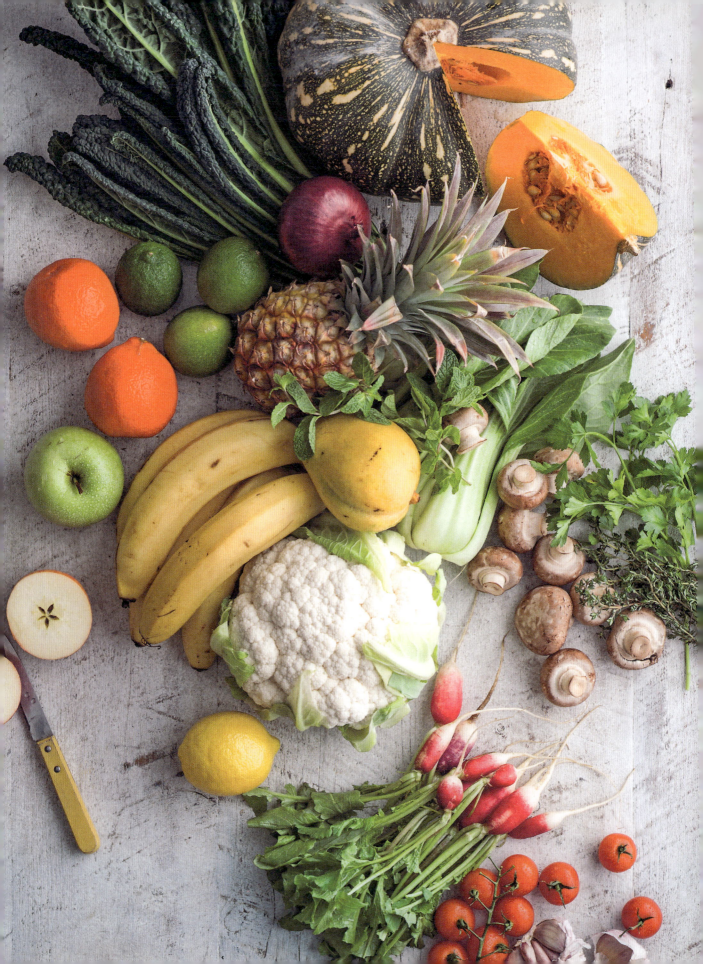

BUILDING ON THE FOUNDATIONS

The Plate is simply a template to get you started. The quantities for each food category are flexible and what you choose to fill each section is up to you. Ask yourself the following questions to help you build on this foundation to create a picture of your family's healthy diet. Bear in mind that everyone's Plate might be a little different, but the foundations are the same.

→ **Does anyone in the family have a food allergy or intolerance?** If one person has a serious food allergy, it might be easier for you all to omit the culprit food altogether, at least in the house. A food intolerance, although often harder to diagnose, is usually less serious so it may not be necessary to eliminate the culprit food or foods from the household.

→ **Are there religious or ethical grounds for exclusion of certain foods or rationale for food combinations?** This includes whether you or someone in your family has chosen to avoid animal foods or to adhere to the dietary rules of a particular faith. These choices should incorporate good nutrition.

→ **Are there cultural associations your family has with certain foods that you would like to honour?** Or are there foods that are more familiar to you based on your background and ancestry? For example, I grew up in Scotland where potatoes were a staple – to this day they are a food I love. (And potatoes can be healthy, by the way.) If your family comes from Asia it may be difficult to imagine a diet without rice, or if you're from the Middle East, chickpeas might feature prominently. The truth is that the traditional fare of most countries is pretty healthy – it's the modern, ultra-processed Westernised diet that has been a health disaster. Embrace your cultural associations with food and celebrate them.

→ **What about the likes and dislikes of everyone in the family?** There is not a single food that is essential to a healthy diet. If you or a family member truly dislike something, there are always alternatives. I'll talk about how to deal with fussy eaters later (see page 20), but for now think about having a little respect for the fact that we do have inherent and learned likes and dislikes. Provided another healthy option in the same food category is chosen, then all is well for the family's nutrition. This doesn't mean letting kids avoid eating vegetables! The rule I have always adopted in my house is that the kids have to taste everything on their plate and if they truly don't like it they can leave it. I'll then offer that food again another time. Meanwhile, I have avoided an unhelpful meltdown or standoff at the dinner table.

→ **Don't have the right ingredients in the fridge or pantry?** If you don't have all the ingredients for one of our recipes, relax – just use more of something else. The ingredient list might look long at first glance, but that doesn't mean that the recipe is complicated. Many of our ingredients are fresh herbs or other plant foods – just use the recipe as a guide.

Following the Plate template makes it so easy to design a meal for anyone, no matter what their dietary needs or preferences are.

FROM TODDLERS TO TEENS

When a first baby is born into a family, parents are often highly motivated to be healthier and, of course, all parents want to feed their babies as well as they possibly can. On the other hand, it can feel overwhelming with all sorts of advice (all well meaning but often contradictory) coming from extended family, friends, health professionals and good old 'Dr Google'.

Don't let all of this advice confuse you. I'm going to outline the big picture on what babies need and give you some ideas as to how to integrate your baby into family eating.

Too often I speak to parents who make one meal for the kids and another meal for the adults. The baby or toddler is fed store-bought baby food because it's too hard to make another meal for them. Even worse, sometimes the adults have separate meals because one is on a special diet of some sort. No wonder cooking becomes a chore! The goal is to have your whole family eating a version of the same meal. Aside from the benefits of role-modelling healthy eating and a good relationship with food, this saves time, money and effort.

For example, you might make spaghetti bolognese for the family dinner. Before adding any salt, you remove a little serve for your baby or toddler. You purée, mash or finely chop this to suit the child's age. You make a big salad for the table and then serve up everyone's meal. Active teenagers will need more pasta and sauce to refuel and fill them up, but are still encouraged to have a serve of salad to boost their vegie intake. Mum and dad, having sat at a desk most of the day, have a bigger serve of salad and less pasta. Meanwhile, the toddler can be sitting at the table in a highchair with essentially the same meal, made appropriate for them.

BABIES AND TODDLERS

The first one thousand days of life (from conception to the second birthday) is a golden window of opportunity to set up a child for a healthy life. Think of it as being when the foundations are laid. It's when there is rapid development of the entire body, including the brain, all other organs and, importantly, the systems for immune function, nervous function, metabolism and so on.

This is also the time when the gut microbiome – the bacteria and other microorganisms that inhabit the gut – is established. The gut microbiome plays a key role in the establishment of many of these systems; in particular, the microbiome 'trains' the immune system and is thought to play a role in whether or not allergies, food intolerances and auto-immune problems develop. Ensuring a healthy, plant-rich diet with a diversity of fibre types encourages a healthy, diverse microbiome.

In short, whatever happens during this period can affect the health and wellbeing of a child for the rest of his or her life. That is not meant to alarm you! Rather, I hope it motivates you to get your little ones eating well.

The good news is that you really don't need to cook a separate meal for your toddler!

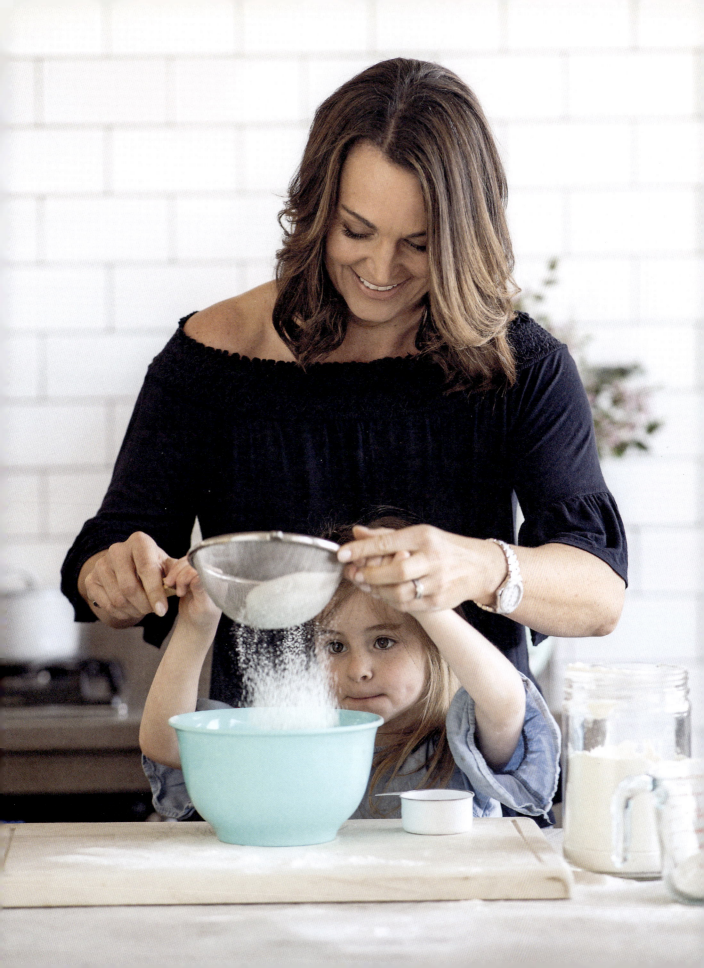

KEY POINTS FOR FEEDING BABIES:

→ **Exclusive breastfeeding is the best way to feed a baby from birth until around 6 months of age.** Breastmilk contains unique carbohydrates that human digestive enzymes cannot break down; they are there specifically to fuel the developing microbiome, which helps babies to develop a strong immune system. Breastmilk also contains antibodies that help the baby fight off harmful bacteria and viruses. As a result, babies who are breastfed have fewer ear infections, fewer coughs and colds, and fewer tummy bugs that cause diarrhoea. They also have fewer allergies and a lower risk of developing asthma. They are more likely to be a healthy weight and into adulthood they have a lower risk of obesity. It's really pretty incredible and shows the importance of the right balance of nutrition in those early months – and mum's body produces it naturally.

→ **There are many situations when breastfeeding is just not possible or too difficult, or, for whatever reason, mum decides it isn't for her and her baby.** In such situations, the next best thing is infant formula. These are improving all the time and, while they cannot exactly match breastmilk, they are a safe, nutritious way to feed your baby. Many now contain prebiotics (the special fibres that feed the microbiome) and probiotics (the 'good' bacteria). Research has shown that the lower-protein formulas that more closely match the protein content of breastmilk are best for babies. Higher-protein formulas tend to make babies gain too much weight and could be a risk for obesity later. Be sure to make up formula according to the packet instructions and use formula alone or combined with breastfeeding to around 6 months.

→ **Babies are all different, so there is no set time to introduce solids.** However, research shows that the optimal time is somewhere between 5 and 7 months of age. You'll find lots of advice on how to wean your baby in books dedicated to the topic. Overall, think of using whole foods and don't succumb to thinking you need to buy specific baby foods. Baby rice, for example, is a modern, highly processed food. You are much better off puréeing whole foods, such as cooked brown rice with lots of vegies. Babies who are over 6 months need a source of iron, so feeding them puréed meat meals is a good idea. There's no need to serve each food individually – that is old-fashioned advice. Puréeing family meals, ensuring there is no added salt or sugar, will make things easier for you and ensure best nutrition for your baby.

→ **If you are breastfeeding and are keen and able to continue to do so, it's a good idea while weaning, particularly when you're introducing potentially allergenic foods such as eggs, nuts and fish.** For all babies, it is good to introduce such foods, and research shows that avoiding them until later in childhood can actually increase the risk of allergy. If you are at all worried, speak to your GP or other healthcare professional.

→ **Get babies and toddlers eating vegies early to make them a normal part of their meals.** You also want to get them eating other whole plant foods, including wholegrains. Many parents think they should give white bread and rice to babies and toddlers and avoid the wholegrain versions. This is absolutely not true! Get them used to real, whole food from the start.

→ **If you are vegetarian or vegan and want to raise your child this way, I urge you to consult a dietitian to help you ensure a nutritionally adequate diet.** Babies and children have relatively high requirements for certain key nutrients, including iron, zinc, calcium and long-chain omega-3 fats, that are absorbed best from animal products. It's possible to meet these requirements with plant foods, but it takes more careful planning. Get help to make sure you achieve it.

→ **One of my pet hates is seeing toddlers who are still eating puréed foods that have come from a pouch-style packet or, worse still, sucking the food themselves from the spout and still drinking from a bottle.** It's crucial that babies and toddlers move through stages of texture with foods because this helps them to develop the muscles they need for chewing, as well as the coordination and the acceptance of a diversity of tastes. As they are ready, move them from puréed to mashed to increasingly textured foods. By 12 months of age, babies should be eating most family meals, with small adaptations where necessary.

→ **The only drinks that should be given to babies and toddlers are water and milk, and only water at mealtimes so they don't fill up on milk.** Don't give them artificially sweetened drinks, including those that are sweetened with stevia or other so-called 'natural' sweeteners, and never give them fruit juices or soft drinks. Use full-fat milk and other full-fat dairy products. If dairy must be avoided, ensure that you use a calcium-fortified, nutritionally adequate alternative such as soy.

Remember, the food and drink that babies and toddlers have can affect their health and wellbeing for life. It's worth putting in the effort to set up good eating habits and get them off to the very best start.

PRE-SCHOOLERS

This is often the age when children get fussy with their food. In part, this is due to them recognising that it is something they have control over. They can refuse to eat something and set up demands for foods they particularly like. It is absolutely crucial to lay down good eating foundations at this point and not give in by always cooking the meals that you know they like. How are they to ever expand their taste palate if they are only ever given 'kids' meals'?

That said, some children really do have problems with expanding their food repertoire. Children who have been hospitalised or had major health issues during the weaning and toddler stages can have delayed or impaired development of the muscles and coordination required to eat, or they might have gut problems, often associated with conditions such as autism. Seek professional help if your child's food fussiness seems extreme or you are struggling to manage it.

It's common for pre-schoolers to become fussy with food, but it's crucial to set good foundations.

For most kids, the best approach to mealtimes is to be calm and consistent and, above all, try to make them a happy time of the day. That's easier said than done, I know – Mel and I have both found ourselves yelling at our kids to eat the food we have lovingly prepared! But that approach never works and only ends up with everyone being upset, most of all you.

IMPORTANT NUTRITIONAL ASPECTS FOR PRE-SCHOOLERS:

→ **Kids at this age want to have some control, so give them some – within your boundaries.** Try offering a choice between two healthy foods or meals. For example, shall we have broccoli or carrots with dinner? Would you like sliced apple or pear for afternoon tea?

→ **Take your kids grocery shopping with you when you are not in a hurry.** Discuss the fresh produce on display, get them to feel various fruits and vegies so they become more familiar with them, and let them help to choose what you buy.

→ **Start to talk to them in age-appropriate language about why it is important to eat healthy foods.** I spoke to my kids about brain food (tucking into their salmon), muscle food (protein-rich foods) and, their favourite, bottom food (fibre-rich foods like beans). I once told my son that if he ate beetroot it would make his poo purple. He gobbled it up and immediately ran from the table. I then heard him yelling from the bathroom that it hadn't worked! He did, of course, have to give it a little more time, but that led to a discussion on digestion and what happens in your tummy when you eat.

→ **Continue to only give them water or milk to drink, and only water with meals.** Make water the normal drink to reach for when they are thirsty.

→ **The rule I have always adopted in my house is that kids must try everything on their plate, but if they taste it and truly don't like it, they can leave it.** However, there are no replacement meals. Dinner is dinner and if they don't eat it, there's nothing else. I didn't do the old 'you don't get dessert if you don't eat your main meal'. That teaches them that the main meal is not nearly so nice and dessert is where the fun is! Instead, ensure dessert is almost always healthy – fruit and yoghurt, for example – and don't make it a big deal.

→ **Introduce the concept of 'everyday foods' and 'sometimes foods'.** Some experts recommend not using the word 'treats' for those sometimes foods and I understand that rationale, but in reality, most families and kids use the term and it makes sense. I use it for foods like lollies or ice cream, but explain that although these foods can bring pleasure, they are not good for them if they have them too often. Hence, they are 'sometimes foods' and the ones that make their bodies healthy and strong are our 'everyday foods'.

→ **At this age, start to teach kids the difference between wanting to eat a food because it's yummy and wanting to eat because you are truly hungry.** It can be helpful to ask them if they are hungry in their tummy or in their head. It might seem silly, but it is a valuable lifelong skill to be able to eat primarily in response to hunger and not for the myriad of other reasons that tempt us.

CONSTIPATION

Constipation is all too common in kids and is related to diet as well as activity levels, as it is in adults. Kids may complain about frequent sore tummies, cramps and perhaps even nausea and generally not feeling well. It's easy to assume that this is a bug or a food intolerance. Parents sometimes try omitting certain foods (commonly gluten and dairy) or suspect that the child just doesn't want to go to school, when in fact the problem is constipation. Foods are unnecessarily cut out and the root cause is not rectified.

Kids who only eat regular white bread, white rice, peeled potatoes, low-fibre cereals, few vegies and no nuts or seeds won't be getting enough fibre to keep their gut moving as it should. Fibre is absolutely key and they need to eat a variety of different types, which are found in whole plant foods. High-fibre foods include wholegrain bread, cereals and grains, fruit and vegies, nuts and seeds, beans and lentils – essentially, all the smart-carb-rich foods on the Plate (pages 8–9).

Physical activity is also very important for keeping the gut moving. Kids who spend too much time watching TV, playing computer games and doing whatever it is they do on their smart phones are more likely to end up with gut issues. A sedentary life leads to a sedentary gut. The physical activity guidelines for kids specify at least an hour of moderate to vigorous exercise every day, as well as several hours of light activities a week.

PRIMARY SCHOOL KIDS

Kids need to learn how to manage their appetite and when to stop eating, rather than to always simply finish the plate – forcing kids to eat everything on the plate teaches them a habit that most adults then struggle to break! I love the Japanese saying 'hara hachi bu'. It means eat until you are about 80 per cent full. That means recognising when you are satisfied rather than completely stuffed. I taught this to my kids at an early age and they still say it to me now when they have had enough to eat.

At this age, kids should be having 4½ to 5 serves a day of vegetables or beans and lentils. Sadly, very few kids are managing this. What's important here are the nutrients, fibre and phytochemicals provided by these foods, but also what kids are eating instead. A lack of vegetables means they are eating too much of other foods.

Step up your language in teaching your kids about good nutrition and why it is important that they eat well. Get them more involved in cooking and preparing meals and make certain they have a healthy lunchbox to take to school. Make healthy eating normal – it's just what you do in your family and not something to make any big deal about. Above all, you want mealtimes to be a pleasant, enjoyable time of the day, rather than a source of conflict and stress for everyone.

HOW DO I GET MY KIDS TO EAT THEIR VEGIES?

→ **Make vegies tasty!** Cooking with flavour helps to make vegies tastier and more appealing. Roast them in balsamic vinegar and extra virgin olive oil, stir-fry them with some fresh herbs and spices, drizzle them with extra virgin olive oil and sprinkle with crushed nuts, mash them with potatoes or beans to make a healthier 'mash' or toss them in extra virgin olive oil and air-fry to make your own vegie chips. Or why not make a traditional béchamel sauce to pour over a lovely tray of mixed steamed vegies? Sprinkle some grated cheese over the top and the kids (and adults) will almost certainly ask for seconds!

→ **Make vegies an integral part of the meal rather than always having them on the side.** Finely dice or grate vegies and add them to your curries, casseroles, burgers, meatballs and pasta or rice dishes. Try a few different vegetarian recipes where vegies are the hero of the dish, such as a vegie lasagne or vegie and bean casserole.

→ **There's nothing wrong with a traditional meat, potatoes and three veg meal – just be sure not to overcook the vegies!** If you're cooking vegetables from frozen, remember that they're already cooked and really only need thawing and heating through. The best way to cook fresh vegies in order to preserve their taste and nutrition is to steam, microwave, roast or stir-fry them.

→ **Get vegies into at least two meals a day.** If you only give your kids vegies at dinner, you'll never meet the recommended serves a day. When you have time to cook breakfast, try making an omelette with mushrooms and spinach. Bake a vegetable frittata that can be eaten hot at home or go cold into the lunchbox. Pop some salad vegies into their sandwich or wrap or put them separately as batons with a hummus dip.

→ **Beans and lentils count towards daily vegie serves and kids often love these foods.** What about baked beans on a toasted wholemeal English muffin, topped with a little grated cheese for breakfast? Try serving a lentil, bean or minestrone soup for lunch. Or a dinner of spaghetti bolognese with added borlotti beans, or a lentil dhal with brown rice and a vegetable-rich mild curry.

→ **Make a big pot of vegie or legume soup.** Blend the soup to a smooth texture if the kids don't like it lumpy or with 'bits'.

Talk about vegies in a positive way and set a good example by eating plenty of them yourself.

FUSSY EATERS

Fussy eaters can drive you mad and make family dinners a battleground. Above all, don't let that happen. Keep your cool and always try to make mealtimes a pleasant part of the day.

It's very normal for younger kids to go through a fussy stage. It is actually part of normal development to be wary of new foods – kids have to learn that these are not harmful. They do that by seeing their parents and other people they trust eating the food. They are then more likely to try it for themselves. Therein lies the first point – you have to be a good role-model!

Kids also have more sensitive tastebuds than adults and many foods taste stronger or differently to how adults taste them. Cruciferous vegetables such as brussels sprouts and cabbage are good examples. These can taste quite bitter to kids and they are more likely to reject them than a sweeter vegetable, such as carrots. That doesn't mean you don't serve them! Mixing them with a sweeter vegie can make them more acceptable, or try adding a sauce to balance the flavour.

TIPS FOR FAMILIES WITH A FUSSY EATER:

→ **If they won't eat the meal, don't bow to pressure to give them something you know they will eat instead.** That simply reinforces that they get their own way, making it harder and harder to break the cycle.

→ **Give them some say in what the meal will be.** You might say, 'Shall we have roast chicken tonight or a chicken pasta?', or give them a choice of vegies – 'Would you like carrots or peas with your fish?'

→ **Encourage them to try everything on the plate and, if they have tasted it and really dislike it, they can leave it.** But emphasise that there is nothing else – this is the meal.

→ **It can take up to 20 times for a child to accept a new food, so don't give up after one rejection.** Try giving them a new food alongside familiar foods. If it is rejected, then don't make a fuss. Simply try again another time.

→ **Rest assured that your child will not starve.** We spend so much time when they are babies trying to ensure they have a full tummy so they sleep better that we often find it hard to let that go as they get older. If they don't eat at one meal, you can bet they will at the next when they are then really hungry. Just be sure you don't allow them to fill up on snacks in between.

TEENAGERS

The teenage years are critical for growth and development. Boys in particular tend to go through a very rapid growth spurt, while the growth for girls may be more consistent. Teenagers have increased needs for most nutrients, including protein to support that growth, vitamins and minerals. They also need more energy, particularly if they are doing a lot of sport.

At the same time, teenagers may be making more of their own food choices when they're out and about without you, or at home helping themselves from the kitchen. They may be tempted by sports drinks and supplements if training hard, or fast foods and energy-dense snacks that don't give them the nutrition they need.

Teenagers may become more body conscious, and helping them to have a healthy body image is important. They may be concerned that they are overweight or underweight and this can lead to them falling for the lure of fad diets or even eliminating certain foods or whole food groups, with nutritional and potentially mental health consequences. See page 25 for more on creating a healthy relationship with food.

WAYS TO ENCOURAGE HEALTHY EATING IN TEENS:

→ **Stock the kitchen with plenty of healthy eating options that are easy for them to grab or make.** Healthy muesli, oat or nut bars to eat on the run; ready-cut vegie sticks to have with nut butter, hummus or avocado; wholegrain bread they can make into sandwiches or toast and top with nut butter, avocado, banana or beans and cheese; a variety of wholegrain breakfast cereals for quick breakfasts and snacks. And teach them how to make a smoothie!

→ **Make eating dinner together as a family a priority.** Teenagers who eat with the family do tend to have healthier diets. They might appear to rebel, but in fact you remain a role-model, whether they seem to be paying attention to you or not! Keep family healthy eating as the goal for everyone rather than focusing on individuals and you will all benefit.

→ **Continue to give them a packed lunch, particularly if they can eat outside the school or if the school canteen is not as healthy as you would like.** They can, of course, start making lunch themselves, but keep an eye on what they pack! Be sure to give them enough to eat, particularly if they have sport or other activities after school. They might need an extra sandwich or snack.

→ **Talk about why eating well is important.** They will hopefully be learning at least basic nutrition at school, but expand on this at home. Discuss why fad diets and celebrity-endorsed dietary trends are potentially dangerous. If you're not sure of the facts or arguments, find reputable online sources of information to help. Teach teens to get all their information, including nutrition and diet information, from qualified reputable sources, and how to tell the difference between reliable and unreliable sources.

→ **Teach them how to cook at least the basics, and if they show interest they might surprise you and become more adventurous.** How wonderful if one of your teens starts to produce the family meal on occasion!

→ **Talk to them about the dangers of social media and encourage them to unfollow anyone that makes them feel bad about their own body or how they look.** Make sure they realise that many of the images of bodies they see are altered and filtered so much that they don't reflect reality.

→ **Make sure you are a positive body role-model.** As a family, talk about what your bodies do rather than what they look like. Never comment on other people's weight. It's so common for people to reward people with a comment such as: 'You've lost weight, you look great!' All that does is reinforce the message that thinner is more attractive. Besides, the weight loss might be due to stress or illness. Keep the family focus firmly on health from the inside out.

→ **Make it clear that it is not OK to tease anyone about their weight, either within the family or with their peers.**

→ **Encourage them to have pride in their abilities as this is where they will build good self-esteem.** In turn, good self-esteem is what will help teenagers to deflect any negative messages about body image.

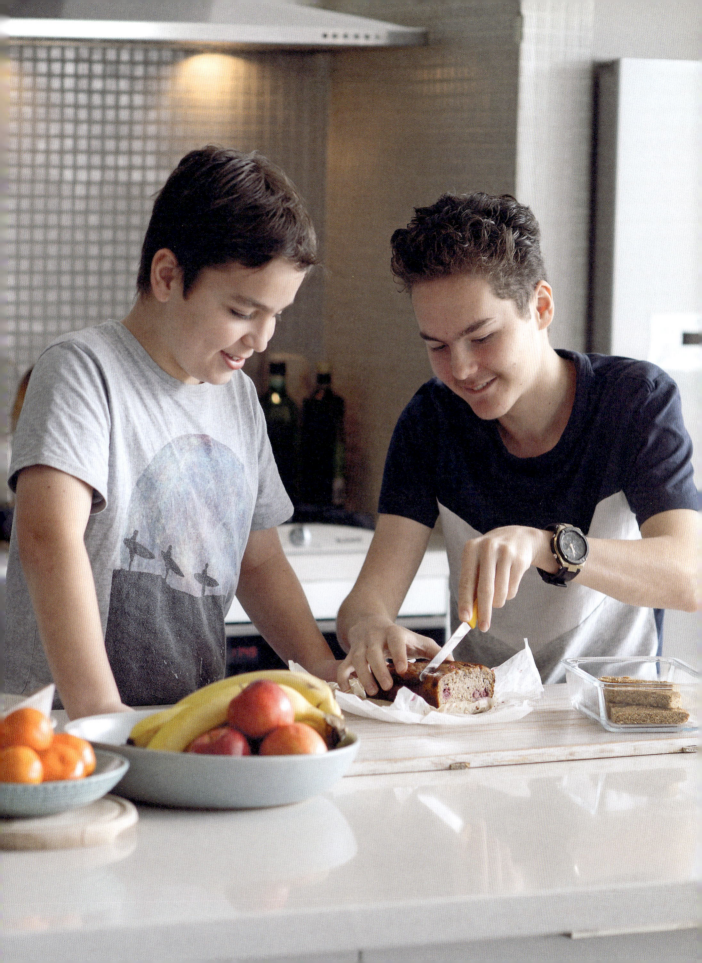

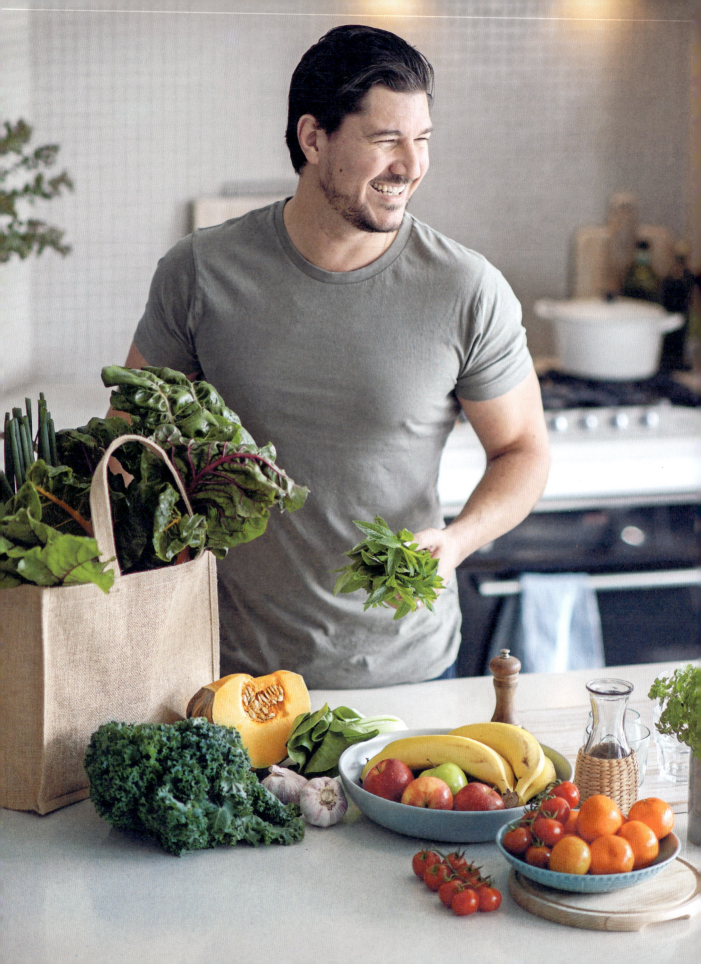

CREATING A HEALTHY RELATIONSHIP WITH FOOD

EMBRACE FAMILY MEALTIMES

Eating as a family as often as possible is a great idea on all sorts of levels. Modern life can be hectic, with everyone on different schedules, making family dinners around the table more difficult. But I strongly encourage you to make it happen as often as you can.

Eating together at the table encourages positive eating habits, particularly if you reinforce them. It's an opportunity to teach and model to kids why nutrition is important and what healthy eating is. So be sure you're being a good role-model – if you don't eat your vegies, neither will they!

Eating at the table encourages mindful eating, whereas eating on the run or in front of the TV creates mindless eating, when overeating is much more likely. Plus, it's much easier to monitor what and how your kids are eating when you all do it together.

Dinner is the meal families are most likely to spend together, but on the weekend it could be brunch or Sunday lunch. Embrace these traditions and keep the fun and social aspects of mealtimes alive. It's all part of creating or maintaining a healthy relationship with food for ourselves and our kids.

SIT DOWN TO EAT

Even when it's not possible to have the whole family together for a meal, encourage everyone to eat at the table or kitchen bench. Giving priority to meals is part of recognising how important feeding ourselves is. It shows respect to food, rather than absentmindedly stuffing whatever is available, or we take fancy to, down our throats.

There will inevitably be times when eating on the run is preferable to not eating at all – at least for the kids. Adults can generally go for much longer without food than kids can, especially younger kids. But even adults might find themselves needing to eat on the way to work or between meetings. Having a stash of healthier packaged snacks in your pantry and a few meals that are quick to throw together, or snacks that are easy to eat in the car, or on the run, will at least ensure good nutrition.

There are so many physical, social, mental and emotional benefits to sitting down to a meal as a family.

SPEAK POSITIVELY ABOUT BODIES

To create a healthy relationship with food, you need to also have a healthy, positive relationship with your own body. If a mother is consistently belittling her own body, asking if her thighs or bum look big, frequently jumping onto the latest fad diet or using unhealthy means to try to lose weight, then the kids, especially daughters, will quickly learn to assess their own bodies in the same way and might start to mimic these behaviours.

Men are also coming under increasing pressure to conform to an ideal of what is considered attractive and boys are acutely aware of this. They might be self-conscious about their own bodies as a result and this can lead to unhealthy eating behaviours.

We can't shield our kids entirely from society's pressures, but we can help them to build a healthy relationship with food and view their own bodies positively. This will, in turn, make them more resilient to those pressures.

Always speak in a positive way about your own body and anyone else's body. This doesn't mean that you have to ignore the issue of overweight and obesity, or underweight for that matter. But it does mean we don't describe or define people by their body shape. Bodies come in all shapes and sizes and the goal is to help your body be the healthiest it can be. Explain this to your kids, teaching them that some people are short, some tall, some have smaller bodies and others larger bodies. What is important for all of us is to look after our bodies to ensure they are as healthy as possible and that is why we need to eat well, do enough activity and exercise, get enough sleep and manage our stress levels.

WHAT IF YOUR CHILD IS OVERWEIGHT?

There are medical criteria for assessing whether both children and adults are overweight, but the truth is that you probably know. The important point is that by the time they go to school, they probably do too. There is nothing to be gained and much to lose by labelling a child as overweight.

This doesn't mean that you can't talk to them about their weight. In fact, it's generally a good thing that you do, otherwise they could bottle up their own thoughts and feelings on the topic. Place your focus firmly on health rather than aesthetics.

Encourage them to think about what their body can do, not what it looks like. Talk about other bodies in the same way, including your own. Encourage them to eat well so that their brain is firing in class, making them better at their school work, or that their muscles are well-fuelled, allowing them to perform at their best on the sports field.

Regardless of whether the whole family is overweight or just one child, look to make changes to the way everybody eats. Eating well and living a healthy lifestyle is about much more than weight control. Weight does not tell you how healthy a person is. Make sure no one in the family is singled out and instead adopt a healthy eating policy for the whole family. Be active as a family and, above all, make sure that the adults in the household are being good role-models for healthy living.

Kids have the advantage that they are still growing, so a shift towards healthier eating and building healthy lifestyle behaviours is all many of them need as they grow into their weight. If you're at all worried about your child's weight and feel you need more help, speak with your GP or a dietitian. There are many family programs that can help.

WHAT IF YOUR CHILD IS UNDERWEIGHT?

The first step is to ascertain whether your child really is underweight and whether it is something that needs further exploration. Some kids are just naturally thinner, just as other kids are naturally bigger. If the child is eating healthily and is active daily with no related health problems, then relax and continue to help them build a healthy relationship with food and with their own body.

If your child is truly underweight, observe their eating habits and consider whether these are contributing. See your GP for a medical checkup and to diagnose common nutritional deficiencies if you are worried.

If the problem is simply one of not eating enough, try not to resort to giving them unhealthy, nutrient-poor foods and drinks simply to get them to eat. All kids, regardless of their size, need nutritious foods to support their growth and development. Plus, you want to help them build healthy habits that last a lifetime. Healthy eating should be their default, being what they are used to at home.

Instead, ensure you give them plenty of nutrient- and energy-dense foods, particularly if they have a small appetite and can't eat much in a single sitting. Foods that are rich in healthy fats are ideal – use full-fat dairy products, drizzle their pasta and vegies with extra virgin olive oil, spread avocado on their toast and in sandwiches and wraps, and use nut butters in smoothies, on toast or crackers, or spread it on celery. Even if they're not allowed to take nut products to school, they should absolutely be having nuts at home (allergies excepted, of course). And try giving a few more nutritious snacks so that they eat more regularly, with the caveat that you want them to be hungry by mealtimes, so be careful with the timing of snacks.

Finally, make sure they are not filling up on milk or juice and then not eating their meals as a result. Some kids are lazier with chewing and eating and simply have less interest in food. If you give them the easy option of filling their tummy with liquids, many will take it!

As parents, you are the most important role-models for your children in terms of a healthy lifestyle.

IDEAS FOR GETTING KIDS INTERESTED IN FOOD AND COOKING:

→ **Get them involved!** Cooking and preparing food are life skills that will benefit kids in the future, but even younger kids can help with simple jobs to help you get meals onto the table.

→ **Allow them to choose between two or three healthy recipes for dinner each week.** If you have more than one child, then each one gets a night to choose. Then make them the sous chef, helping you to prepare and cook the meal. If they have helped cook it, they'll be more interested in eating it.

→ **Kids love to get messy, so don't be too precious about tidiness when they're helping.** They will love getting their (clean!) hands into a meat mixture to make meatballs or burgers, or dipping fish or chicken into flour, egg and breadcrumbs to make homemade fish fingers or schnitzel.

→ **Kids love home baking.** There are plenty of jobs they can do, depending on their age, from sifting flour, to cracking eggs and mixing ingredients. Try making healthy wholegrain muffins, fruit loaf, oat chocolate chip cookies or banana bread that you can then use in their lunchboxes.

→ **Get kids interested in the flavour of food by encouraging them to taste different cuisines, rather than always giving them what you know they like.** Make those meals in the kitchen together and discuss the different spices or herbs used in the dish.

→ **Encourage older kids to make some of their meals for themselves.** Teach teenagers to make scrambled eggs or an omelette, whip up a smoothie or make a baked bean and cheese jaffle. Once they're fairly competent in the kitchen, get them to cook the family meal one night a week. They might just surprise you and rise to the challenge!

→ **Kids will inevitably be keen on making sweet treats and this is fine every now and again.** But they also need to learn the basics. Save the making of sweet treats for perhaps once on the weekend and encourage them to help with main meal preparation as well.

→ **Try growing some of your own food at home and get the kids involved.** You can plant vegies if you have room, or simply a pot of fresh herbs.

→ **Be patient and try to enjoy the process of preparing the meal, rather than rushing them.** Clearly you don't want to get them helping on a night that you really are in a rush unless they are truly helpful. The more you get them helping, the better help they will actually be.

→ **Resist the temptation to always step in and do things for them.** Any new skill takes time to get right and cooking is no exception. They may well not chop the onion as finely as you would like or grate the cheese as quickly as you can, but does it really matter for the end result?

→ **Make sure they also help with the cleaning up.** Get kids washing dishes, wiping benches and clearing the table.

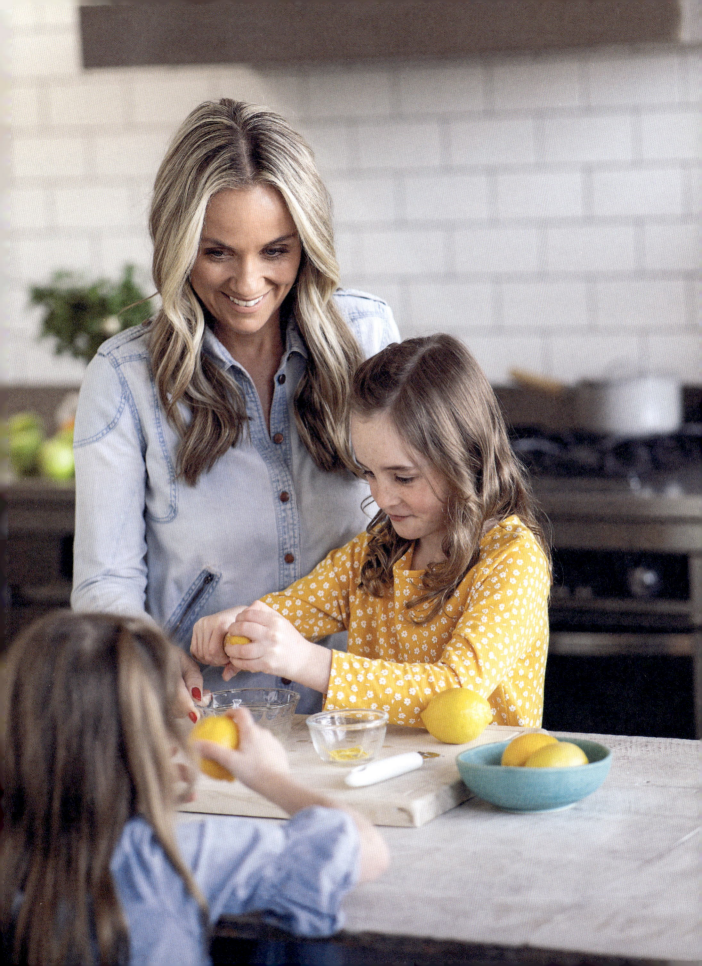

PREPARATION IS THE KEY TO HEALTHY EATING

Never was the motto 'be prepared' more appropriate than when it comes to healthy eating. Make the path easier for everyone to follow and they are more likely to take that route. That's where a little thoughtful preparation comes in. All families are different, with their own favourite meals as well as foods they don't eat (for whatever reason); some families have young children or teenagers, or even elderly parents living with them. The seasonal meal plans on pages 32–35 are designed as a guide to give you an idea of what a week might look like. You can adapt them to suit your individual family.

TIPS FOR SMART MEAL PREPARATION:

→ **When cooking anything that will freeze, cook extra.** While there are some good ready-made meal options out there, commercially produced food prepared en masse just can't compare with a home-cooked meal. Plus, home-cooked meals are mostly easier on the wallet. Bolognese, curries, casseroles, stews and soups generally freeze well. When you know you'll be late home or won't feel like cooking, transfer one of these dishes to the fridge the night before to give it time to thaw, and dinner will be a cinch.

→ **When cooking wholegrains such as brown or black rice, quinoa, barley or wholemeal couscous, cook more than you need for that meal.** A grain cooker makes this very easy (see page 233). Divide the extra grains into individual or family-meal size portions, transfer into resealable bags or containers and store in the fridge (if using in the next day or two) or freezer. These are brilliant to thaw and use in salads or buddha-style lunch bowls, or to reheat in the microwave for quick and easy meals.

→ **When you're chopping vegies for dinner, chop extra and store them in resealable containers in the fridge, ready for another meal.**

→ **Chop carrots, celery, cucumber and capsicum into batons and store them in the fridge, ready to serve with a bowl of hummus, guacamole or salsa for afternoon tea or pre-dinner nibbles.** You can also pre-portion vegie batons into containers with a mini pot of hummus to pop into lunchboxes for kids and adults.

→ **Hard-boil a few eggs at the start of the week, write the date on the shell so you remember when you cooked them, pop them in a container and store them in the fridge.** They will last about a week. You can also peel them, place a damp paper towel over the top and store them in a sealed container in the fridge for about 5 days. You then have hard-boiled eggs ready to snack on, to quarter and add to salads, slice as a toast topping, or to mash with a little mayonnaise for sandwich fillings.

→ **When cooking dinner, think about lunch the next day and, where appropriate, make extra to cater for it.**
  → Left-over cooked meat can be sliced ready for sandwiches, rolls, wraps and salad boxes. Even homemade schnitzel, lean burgers and sausages are terrific cold in a sandwich the next day.
  → Some types of fish can also be cooked for using the next day. Salmon, trout and other more robust fish are lovely cold in a sandwich, wrap or salad. There's nothing wrong with using tinned fish, but home-cooked is usually much tastier. I often buy a whole side of salmon rather than buying fillets, cook it for dinner and then I have leftovers to last me for the next couple of days.
  → Other meals are easily reheated in a microwave at work or can be thoroughly reheated at home in the morning and transferred to a thermos container for a portable lunch. My kids love this during the winter months. Pasta bolognese, curries or casseroles with rice or quinoa and soups are all great ideas for the thermos.

→ **When making salad dressing, make up a big batch that will last for several meals.** An oil and vinegar dressing will keep for a couple of weeks and need not be refrigerated. A good basic rule is if all the dressing ingredients came from the pantry, it can be stored in the pantry. In contrast, dressings that are made with any chilled or fresh ingredients such as buttermilk, yoghurt, eggs or fresh herbs should be kept in the fridge and will generally last for 5 to 7 days. (See pages 104–105 for dressings recipes.)

→ **Salad boxes or jars are great to take to work, and these can be prepped on a Sunday for the week ahead.** Keep the dressing in a separate container and add just before eating to ensure the salad stays crisp.

→ **Sunday is also a great day to do a little baking.** Whip up a batch of muffins or cookies that can be used for school lunchboxes over the next few days.

→ **Frozen berries are convenient, just as nutritious as fresh berries, and more economical.** Fresh berries aren't always available and they are often expensive.

→ **Bircher muesli is really, really easy to prepare and makes an awesome breakfast, whether eating at home or on the go.** Invest in a few suitably sized screw-top jars and make up a few serves in one go. Simply combine some rolled oats with your choice of nuts, seeds and dried fruit. Divide among the jars and cover with dairy or plant-based milk. Screw on the tops and store in the fridge for up to 4 to 5 days. On the morning you want to use the muesli, simply add some fresh berries or other fruit and a dollop of yoghurt. You can also use a pre-mixed bircher or natural muesli, but it's generally cheaper to make your own.

→ **There's nothing wrong with letting the kids help themselves to a choice of wholegrain breakfast cereals for breakfast – even if it is every day!** Mornings can be a rush and these cereals make for easy, quick and budget-friendly breakfasts. Encourage the kids to add some fruit, nuts or seeds, and yoghurt.

Family meal plan: SUMMER WEEK 1

	Breakfast	Morning Tea	Lunch	Afternoon Tea	Dinner
Monday	Wholegrain breakfast cereal with fruit, nuts, milk & yoghurt	**Kids:** Sliced pear with chunk of cheese **Adults:** Handful of nuts & berries	**Kids:** Wholemeal wrap with lean roast beef, hummus, lettuce & cucumber **Adults:** Wholemeal wrap with lean roast beef, hummus, lettuce & cucumber	**Kids:** Pot of yoghurt with berries, nuts & pepitas (pumpkin seeds) **Adults:** Wholegrain crackers with guacamole	Vegie Burgers (page 159) in a wholemeal bun or pita bread *Prepare overnight oats & pop into fridge*
Tuesday	Overnight Oats with your choice of toppings (page 40)	**Kids:** Baby cucumbers, cherry tomatoes & guacamole **Adults:** Fruit & handful of nuts	**Kids:** Sandwich with tuna, corn, mayonnaise & lettuce **Adults:** Sandwich with tuna & plenty of salad	**Kids:** Wholegrain crackers with cheese & grapes **Adults:** Green smoothie	Lamb Kofta Mezze Plate (page 117)
Wednesday	Overnight Oats with your choice of toppings (page 40)	**Kids:** Sliced pear with chunk of cheese **Adults:** Carrot & celery sticks with guacamole	**Kids:** Wholegrain wrap with left-over lamb koftas, hummus, lettuce & tzatziki **Adults:** Wholegrain wrap with left-over lamb koftas, hummus, lettuce & tzatziki	**Kids:** Bag of popcorn **Adults:** Mixed berries, nuts & dark chocolate	Semolina-crusted Sweet Potato (page 198) with grilled or barbecued pork fillet & a mixed salad *Cook extra pork for lunch tomorrow*
Thursday	Wholegrain breakfast cereal with fruit, nuts, milk & yoghurt	**Kids:** Baby cucumbers, cherry tomatoes & guacamole **Adults:** Fruit & handful of nuts	**Kids:** Sandwich with left-over pork, grated apple, lettuce & cream cheese **Adults:** Salad bowl/jar with mixed vegies, left-over pork & a side of wholegrain bread	**Kids:** Wholegrain crackers & celery sticks with nut butter **Adults:** Green smoothie	Gado Gado Vegetables with Tempeh (page 168)
Friday	Boiled eggs with avocado on wholegrain toast	**Kids:** Pot of yoghurt with berries **Adults:** Berry & yoghurt-based smoothie	**Kids:** Wholegrain wrap with feta, hummus, cucumber, grated carrot, lettuce & tomato **Adults:** Salad bowl/jar with mixed vegies, feta & tinned beans or chickpeas	**Kids:** Wholemeal fruit muffin **Adults:** Mixed nuts with dates or dried figs	Potato & Green Bean Salad with Olive Caper Dressing (page 201) with grilled or barbecued salmon fillets **Dessert:** Strawberries with ice cream
Saturday	Jaffle with your choice of filling (page 42)	Breakfast Smoothie (page 39)	Beef, Beet and Zucchini Burgers (page 160) in wholemeal buns with salad vegies, relish & cheese	Grazing platter for everyone to share with your choice of nuts, wholegrain corn chips, vegie sticks, hummus, guacamole & tzatziki	Barbecued Chilli Prawns (page 155) with yoghurt-dressed coleslaw & wholemeal tortillas **Dessert:** Yoghurt Labneh Cheesecake (page 213)
Sunday	Fried Eggs with Haloumi & Grated Vegetables (page 47)	Fruit	Salad bowl with tinned tuna & tinned beans with a dressing from pages 104–105, with crusty wholegrain bread	Baked Muesli Bar (page 74) *Store the left-overs in an airtight container to use during the week*	Barbecued Chilli Lime Chicken (page 163) with potato chips (leave skin on, toss in extra virgin olive oil & bake or air-fry) with salad

Teenagers and more active kids may need more food than given above. Add fruit, yoghurt or additional healthy snacks as required.

Family meal plan: SUMMER WEEK 2

	Breakfast	Morning Tea	Lunch	Afternoon Tea	Dinner
Monday	Wholegrain toast with your choice of toppings (pages 60–61)	**Kids:** Pot of yoghurt with passionfruit **Adults:** Fruit & handful of nuts	**Kids:** Sandwich with left-over chicken, avocado, lettuce, cheese & relish **Adults:** Salad bowl/jar of mixed vegies	**Kids:** Baked Muesli Bar (page 74) **Adults:** Green smoothie	Four-mince Bolognese (page 108) with pasta & a green salad *Freeze left-overs for Saturday dinner*
Tuesday	Wholegrain toast with your choice of toppings (pages 60–61)	**Kids:** Baked Muesli Bar (page 74) **Adults:** Handful of nuts	**Kids:** Sandwich with tinned or hot-smoked salmon, cream cheese & lettuce **Adults:** Salad bowl/jar with hot-smoked salmon, corn or beans & vegies	**Kids:** Sliced apple with chunk of cheese **Adults:** Sliced apple with chunk of cheese	Tofu stir-fry with plenty of vegies, served with steamed black rice *Cook extra rice for lunch tomorrow*
Wednesday	Boiled eggs with avocado & tomato on wholegrain toast	**Kids:** Pot of yoghurt with berries **Adults:** Fruit with Greek-style yoghurt	**Kids:** Sandwich with hummus, cheese, lettuce & grated carrot **Adults:** Salmon, Fennel, Kale & Black Rice Salad Jar (page 90)	**Kids:** Bag of popcorn **Adults:** Handful of nuts	Fish Tacos (page 140) *Cook extra fish for lunch tomorrow*
Thursday	Wholegrain breakfast cereal with fruit, nuts, milk & yoghurt	**Kids:** Sliced apple with chunk of cheese **Adults:** Wholegrain crackers with cheese & cucumber	**Kids:** Wholegrain wrap with left-over fish, lettuce, cucumber & avocado **Adults:** Salad bowl/jar with left-over fish & tinned mixed beans	**Kids:** Carrot & celery sticks with hummus **Adults:** Carrot & celery sticks with hummus	Soy Ginger Chicken (page 132) *Cook extra chicken for lunch tomorrow*
Friday	Wholegrain toast with your choice of toppings (pages 60–61)	**Kids:** Pot of yoghurt with berries **Adults:** Fruit with Greek-style yoghurt	**Kids:** Sandwich with left-over chicken, avocado, lettuce & grated carrot **Adults:** Broccolini, Chicken & Rocket Salad (page 96)	**Kids:** Mixed nuts & dates **Adults:** Handful of nuts	Fish Burgers with Coleslaw (page 149)
Saturday	Poached eggs with sautéed mushrooms, wilted spinach, steamed asparagus, avocado & wholegrain toast	Cocoa Banana Protein Shake (page 73)	Chicken Cobb salad with Blue Ranch Dressing (page 102)	Yoghurt with berries & nuts	Left-over bolognese (from Monday), pasta & a green salad **Dessert:** Fruit salad with ice cream
Sunday	Boiled Eggs with Middle Eastern Breakfast Plate (page 48)	Fruit	Broccoli Kale Pesto & Mozzarella Toastie (page 170)	Banana Acai Choc Popsicles (page 209)	Tamari Lamb Skewers (page 152), wholemeal pita or tortillas & a yoghurt-based coleslaw

Teenagers and more active kids may need more food than given above. Add fruit, yoghurt or additional healthy snacks as required.

Family meal plan: WINTER WEEK 1

	Breakfast	Morning Tea	Lunch	Afternoon Tea	Dinner
Monday	Rolled oat porridge topped with berries, Greek-style yoghurt, nuts & a drizzle of maple syrup	**Kids:** Popcorn & sliced apple with chunk of cheese **Adults:** Fruit & handful of nuts	**Kids:** Sandwich with tuna, corn, mayonnaise & lettuce **Adults:** Tamarind Lentil Soup (page 82)	**Kids:** Vegie Ricotta Muffin (page 78) **Adults:** Wholegrain crackers, cheese, sliced cucumber & tomato	Mexican Spiced Stuffed Capsicums (page 167) *Cook extra for lunch tomorrow*
Tuesday	Boiled eggs with avocado on wholegrain toast	**Kids:** Vegie Ricotta Muffin (page 78) **Adults:** Berries & Greek-style yoghurt, topped with nuts	**Kids:** Wholegrain wrap with grated cheese, lettuce, tomato (seeds removed) & relish **Adults:** Left-over Mexican Spiced Stuffed Capsicums	**Kids:** Banana, berries, nuts & yoghurt **Adults:** Green smoothie	Coconut Fish Fingers with Sweet Potato Fries (page 145) & a green salad
Wednesday	Wholegrain breakfast cereal with fruit, nuts, milk & yoghurt	**Kids:** Brown rice crackers with cheese **Adults:** Handful of nuts	**Kids:** Sandwich with egg, mayonnaise & lettuce **Adults:** Super-quick Zucchini Soup (page 81), wholegrain bread & cheese	**Kids:** Muesli bar **Adults:** Carrot & celery sticks with hummus	Chicken Schnitzel (page 125) with steamed broccolini & mash made from potato, cauliflower & parsnip *Cook extra for lunch tomorrow*
Thursday	Poached Eggs with Baked Beans on Muffins (page 52)	**Kids:** Bag of popcorn & mandarin **Adults:** Berries, yoghurt & chia seeds	**Kids:** Wholegrain wrap with left-over chicken schnitzel, hummus, grated carrot & lettuce **Adults:** Wholegrain wrap with left-over chicken schnitzel, hummus, grated carrot & lettuce	**Kids:** Muesli bar **Adults:** Green smoothie	Tuna Chilli Spaghetti (page 139) with a simple green salad *Cook extra for lunch tomorrow*
Friday	Rolled oat porridge topped with berries, Greek-style yoghurt, nuts & a drizzle of maple syrup	**Kids:** Brown rice crackers with cheese **Adults:** Apple	**Kids:** Sandwich with tinned or hot-smoked salmon, cream cheese & lettuce **Adults:** Left-over Tuna Chilli Spaghetti with a handful of baby spinach	**Kids:** Carrot & celery sticks with hummus **Adults:** Carrot & celery sticks with hummus	Roasted Vegetables with Sriracha Tahini Yoghurt (page 195) served with steak
Saturday	Jaffle with your choice of filling (page 42)	Cocoa Banana Protein Shake (page 73)	Quinoa Nasi Goreng (page 185)	Grazing platter for everyone to share with your choice of nuts, wholegrain corn chips, vegie sticks, hummus, guacamole & tzatziki	Pizza (pages 188–193) with a selection of toppings for everyone to make their own, served with a rocket & spinach salad
Sunday	Omelette with your choice of filling (page 51) with wholegrain toast & avocado	Fruit salad with Greek-style yoghurt	Tamarind Lentil Soup (page 82)	Banana Raspberry Nut Loaf (page 77) *Store the left-overs in the fridge for during the week*	Simple Roast Chicken & Veg (page 128) **Dessert:** Maple-baked Banana with Homemade Custard (page 220)

Teenagers and more active kids may need more food than given above. Add fruit, yoghurt or additional healthy snacks as required.

Family meal plan: WINTER WEEK 2

	Breakfast	Morning Tea	Lunch	Afternoon Tea	Dinner
Monday	Rolled oat porridge topped with berries, Greek-style yoghurt, nuts & a drizzle of maple syrup	**Kids:** Sliced apple with chunk of cheese **Adults:** Handful of nuts	**Kids:** Sandwich with left-over roast chicken, avocado, lettuce, grated carrot & chutney **Adults:** Miso soup & sushi	**Kids:** Banana Raspberry Nut Loaf (page 77) **Adults:** Apple	Mediterranean Chicken (page 131)
Tuesday	Boiled eggs with avocado on wholegrain toast	**Kids:** Bag of popcorn & mandarin **Adults:** Carrot & celery sticks with hummus	**Kids:** Sandwich with left-over roast chicken, avocado & lettuce **Adults:** Left-over Mediterranean Chicken	**Kids:** Vegie Ricotta Muffin (page 78) **Adults:** Fruit & yoghurt smoothie	Ricotta Zucchini Meatballs in Tomato Sauce with Soft Polenta (page 110) & steamed green vegies
Wednesday	Wholegrain breakfast cereal with fruit, nuts, milk & yoghurt	**Kids:** Baby cucumbers, cherry tomatoes & guacamole **Adults:** Handful of nuts	**Kids:** Wholegrain wrap with sliced left-over meatballs, lettuce & grated cheese **Adults:** Left-over meatballs with polenta	**Kids:** Banana Raspberry Nut Loaf (page 77) **Adults:** Berries with Greek-style yoghurt & chia seeds	Pesto Tofu Scramble (page 171) tossed through pasta & served with a mixed salad
Thursday	Rolled oat porridge topped with berries, Greek-style yoghurt, nuts & a drizzle of maple syrup	**Kids:** Apple & muesli bar **Adults:** Apple & handful of nuts	**Kids:** Wholegrain wrap with sliced hard-boiled egg, lettuce, tomato (seeds removed) & mayonnaise **Adults:** Vegie-based soup with wholegrain bread	**Kids:** Carrot & celery sticks with hummus **Adults:** Tin of tuna with wholegrain crackers	Pumpkin, Chickpea & Fish Curry (page 142) with steamed black rice *Cook extra rice for dessert tomorrow*
Friday	Scrambled eggs with wholegrain toast, avocado & tomato	**Kids:** Baby cucumbers, cherry tomatoes & guacamole **Adults:** Berries with Greek-style yoghurt & nuts	**Kids:** Sandwich with tuna, corn, mayonnaise & lettuce **Adults:** Left-over Fish Curry	**Kids:** Sliced apple with chunk of cheese **Adults:** Carrot & celery sticks with hummus	Roasted Brussels Sprouts with Bulgur and Soy Vinegar (page 199), grilled or barbecued pork fillets, corn on the cob & baked or air-fried potatoes in their skins **Dessert:** Black Rice Pudding (page 210)
Saturday	Wholegrain toast topped with nut butter & sliced strawberries	Cocoa Banana Protein Shake (page 73)	Pop's Grated Vegetable & Chicken Soup (page 85) with wholegrain crusty bread	Wholegrain crackers with cheese & sliced dates or dried figs	Slow-cooked Lamb Shoulder (page 118) with roasted sweet potatoes & steamed greens
Sunday	Banana Blueberry Buckwheat Hotcakes (page 57)	Fruit & handful of nuts	Pop's Grated Vegetable & Chicken Soup (page 85) with wholegrain crusty bread	Vegie Ricotta Muffin (page 78)	Left-over Lamb & Bean Burrito (page 121) with tomato salsa salad & mixed leafy greens **Dessert:** Fruit salad with hazelnuts, lime and chocolate shavings (page 211)

Teenagers and more active kids may need more food than given above. Add fruit, yoghurt or additional healthy snacks as required.

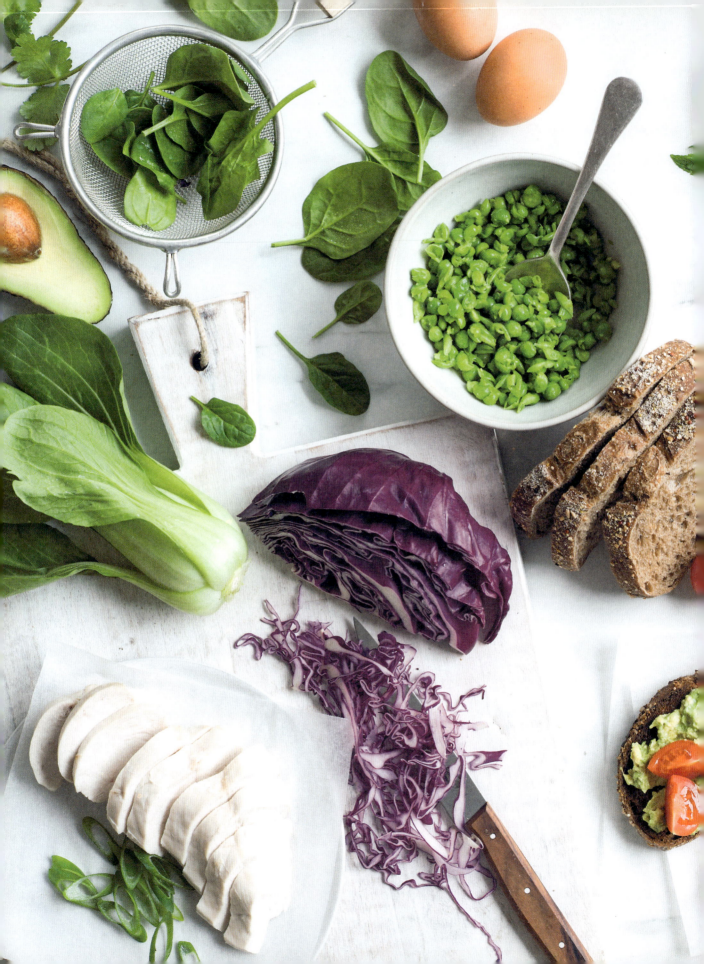

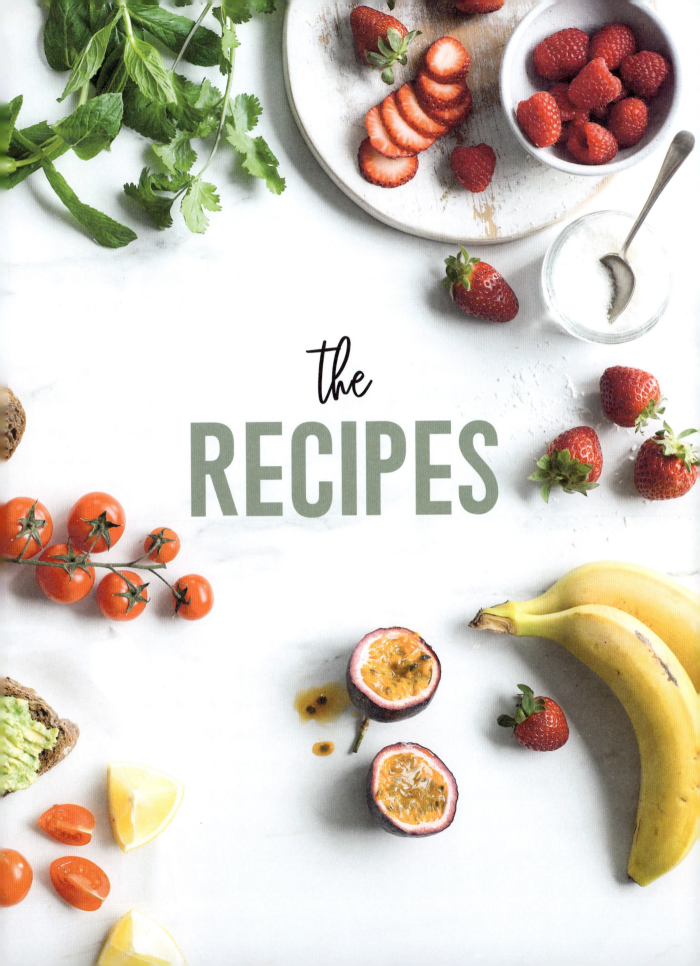

the
RECIPES

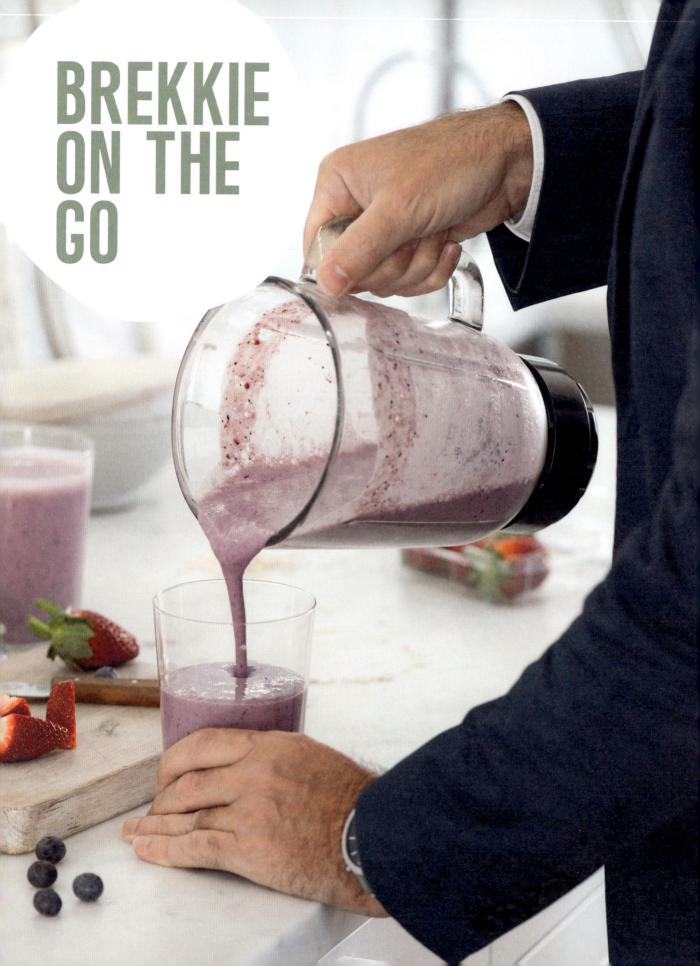

BREKKIE ON THE GO

BREAKFAST SMOOTHIE

PREP TIME: 5 MINUTES 🥤 **COOK TIME: NIL**

As working parents, we know how hard it is to get the family organised, fed and out the door in the mornings, including ourselves! Smoothies are quick to prepare and ideal for breakfast on the run. Simply increase the quantities given to suit the number of serves you need.

SERVES 1

1 cup (250 ml) milk
¼ cup (20 g) rolled oats
30 g raw cashews
½ cup (60 g) frozen mixed berries
½ banana
2 tablespoons Greek-style yoghurt

Put all the ingredients into a blender and blitz until smooth. Pour into a glass or an insulated takeaway cup and run!

TIPS

→ Use any nuts in place of the cashews.
→ This is also a great breakfast to put in an insulated cup for kids to drink after an early morning sport session.
→ The nutritional analyses for our recipes have been calculated using reduced-fat milk and reduced-fat yoghurt, but you can use whatever dairy products your family prefer. Bear in mind that full-fat dairy products are higher in kilojoules.

nutrition per serve   Energy **2030kJ** ‖ Protein **21g** ‖ Fat **21g** (Sat Fat 5g, Poly 3g, Mono 11g)
Carbohydrate **48g** ‖ Fibre **8g**

OVERNIGHT OATS

PREP TIME: 5 MINUTES COOK TIME: **NIL**

When we're rushing to get out the door early, this recipe is a breakfast saviour. Prepared the night before in less than 5 minutes, nothing could be simpler. Increase the quantities and you'll have breakfast covered for a few days. Choose from the topping ideas pictured here, or create your own.

SERVES 4

1 cup (95 g) rolled oats
1 cup (250 ml) milk
1 cup (260 g) Greek-style yoghurt
1 heaped tablespoon chia seeds
2 heaped teaspoons ground cinnamon
2 heaped teaspoons honey

Mix all the ingredients together in a large bowl. Scoop into jars, screw on the lids and refrigerate overnight or until ready to serve.

nutrition per serve

Energy **810kJ** ‖ Protein **10g**
Fat **5g** (Sat Fat 2g, Poly 1.5g, Mono 1.5g)
Carbohydrate **23g** ‖ Fibre **5g**

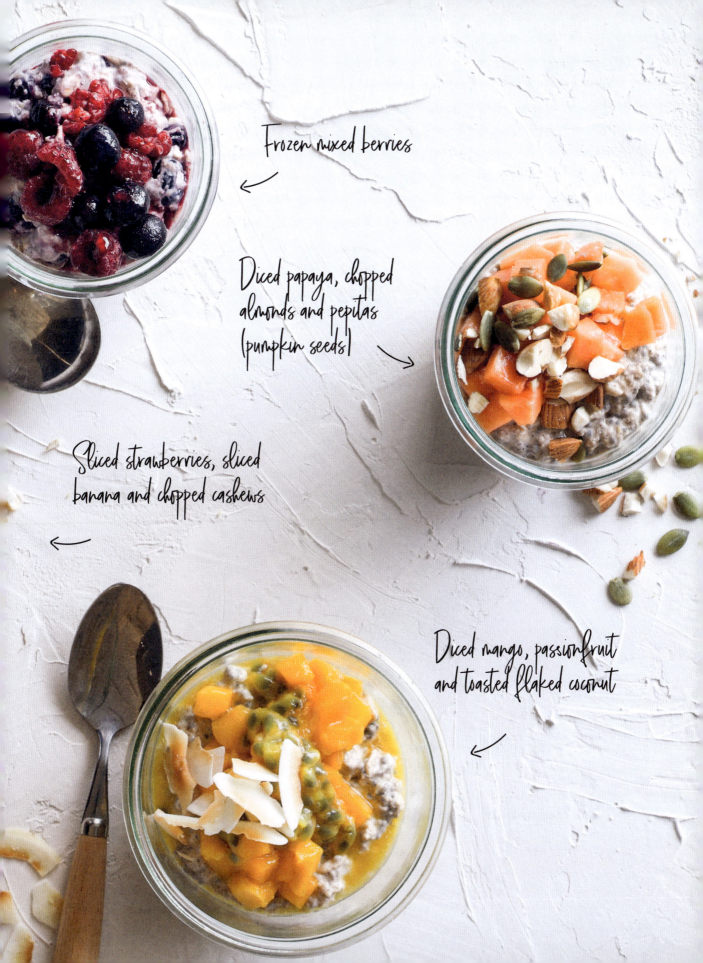

Frozen mixed berries

Diced papaya, chopped almonds and pepitas (pumpkin seeds)

Sliced strawberries, sliced banana and chopped cashews

Diced mango, passionfruit and toasted flaked coconut

JAFFLES

PREP TIME: **5 MINUTES** COOK TIME: **5 MINUTES**

Jaffles are sealed toasted sandwiches, perfect for breakfast or a snack on the run. You can prepare them the night before and have them in the fridge, ready to pop into the jaffle maker before rushing out the door in the morning. Older kids can even make their own jaffles. A baked bean and cheese jaffle is a quick and easy snack when the kids come home starving from sport or school.

SERVES 2

2 tomatoes, sliced
80 g cheddar cheese, sliced
4 slices wholegrain bread

Preheat a non-stick jaffle maker.

Divide the tomato and cheese slices between two of the bread slices, then top with the remaining bread slices.

Carefully place the sandwiches in the jaffle maker. Cook until the bread is golden and the cheese is melted.

Allow the jaffles to cool slightly before serving (the filling can become very hot).

FILLING IDEAS

→ Sliced tomato, cheddar cheese and baby spinach, rocket or flat-leaf parsley
→ Baked beans and cheddar cheese
→ Sautéed mushrooms, baby spinach and grated mozzarella cheese
→ Hummus, left-over roast vegies (such as pumpkin or zucchini), marinated capsicum, pesto and rocket
→ Sliced hard-boiled egg, sliced tomato, avocado and basil
→ Left-over bolognese sauce, baby spinach and cheddar cheese
→ Creamed corn, cheddar cheese and baby spinach

nutrition per serve   Energy **1840kJ** ‖ Protein **21g** ‖ Fat **25g** (Sat Fat 10g, Poly 8g, Mono 6g)
Carbohydrate **26g** ‖ Fibre **8g**

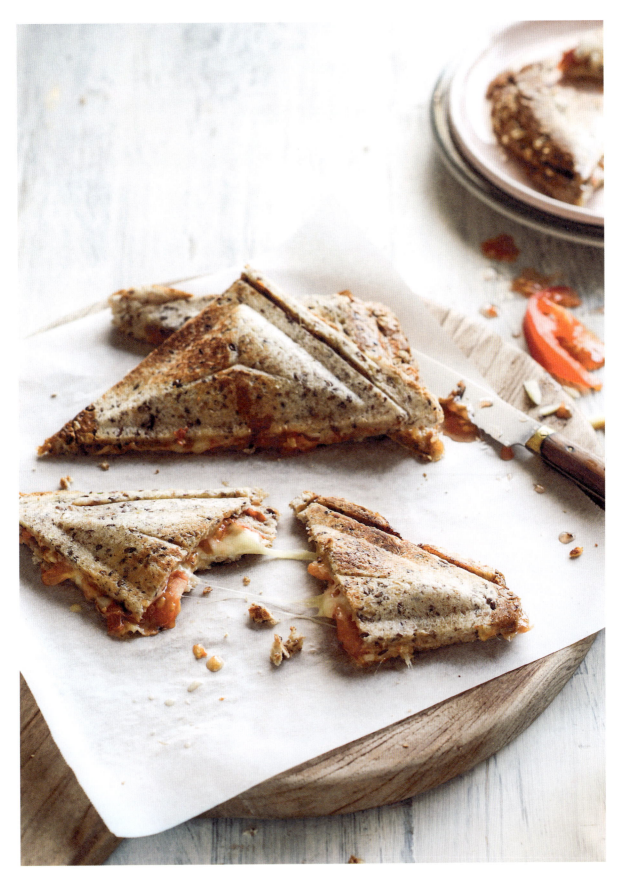

BREAKFAST – THE MOST IMPORTANT MEAL OF THE DAY?

We're so often told that breakfast is the most important meal of the day, and that we should breakfast like a king. But is it actually true?

The truth is that it's your overall diet that's important and so all meals count – breakfast is no more important than any other meal. Some people don't love eating first thing in the morning and that's absolutely fine. There's nothing wrong with waiting to eat.

In fact, there's evidence both for eating and for skipping breakfast in relation to weight control. Studies tend to show that those who eat breakfast are leaner, but a few recent studies show that extending the overnight fast and skipping breakfast helps some people to lose weight, at least in the short term. We really don't know if that is a good strategy in the long run, but since there is growing evidence of the benefits of fasting, this might be an approach that works for you. Others find that eating a healthy breakfast sets them on the right path and they then eat better for the rest of the day. It's also an easy meal to get right as it's usually prepared and eaten at home.

One thing to bear in mind is that breakfast is a key meal for providing fibre, especially cereal fibre, which is very important for gut health and microbiome diversity. If you don't eat breakfast, be sure to get plenty of wholegrain foods into the rest of your day.

When it comes to kids, it's important to ensure they have a good breakfast, at least on school days. There's good evidence that this is key in helping them fire up their brains and for optimal concentration in the classroom. Kids have a smaller capacity to store carbohydrates and other nutrients, so they need to eat more often than adults. Plus, consider that little kids who are in bed earlier have a long time between dinner and breakfast.

If you do struggle to get your kids to eat breakfast, a liquid breakfast can work. Try whipping up a smoothie with milk, yoghurt, fruit, oats and nuts. If they really won't eat anything, give them a more substantial, nutritious snack for morning tea – that smoothie could even go into a thermos flask.

For adults and kids, the quality of the breakfast clearly matters. Fried bacon on white toast slathered with butter and tomato sauce is not the breakfast of champions! Following the Plate model from page 8 is your best guide – see opposite for some ideas.

1. VEGIES AND/ OR FRUIT	2. PROTEIN-RICH FOOD	3. SMART CARBS	4. HEALTHY FATS
WHOLEGRAIN CEREAL WITH FRUIT			
Berries & sliced apple	Milk with Greek-style yoghurt if desired	Wholegrain cereal	Sprinkle of chia seeds
MUESLI WITH BERRIES & YOGHURT			
Blueberries & strawberries	Greek-style yoghurt & a little milk if desired	Natural muesli	Nuts & seeds already present in the muesli
POACHED EGGS ON SOURDOUGH WITH WILTED SPINACH, SAUTÉED MUSHROOMS & GRILLED TOMATO			
Spinach, sautéed mushrooms & grilled tomato	Poached eggs	Wholegrain sourdough toast	Extra virgin olive oil (to cook mushrooms)
BOILED EGGS WITH AVOCADO TOAST SOLDIERS & VEGIE SMOOTHIE			
Green smoothie (with vegies & a little fruit)	Boiled eggs	Wholegrain sourdough toast	Mashed avocado (& Vegemite if you like)
PORRIDGE TOPPED WITH YOGHURT, FRUIT & ROASTED NUTS			
Sliced fruit & berries	Greek-style yoghurt	Porridge made from traditional rolled oats, barley or quinoa	Crushed roasted nuts
SMOKED SALMON, AVOCADO, SPINACH & TOMATO ON TOAST			
Spinach & sliced tomato	Smoked salmon	Wholegrain sourdough toast	Mashed avocado
NUT BUTTER & BANANA ON TOAST WITH A GLASS OF MILK			
Sliced banana	Glass of dairy milk or soy milk	Wholegrain sourdough toast	Peanut butter or other nut butter
MUSHROOM & SPINACH OMELETTE			
Mushrooms & spinach	Eggs	Rye or wholegrain bread	Extra virgin olive oil (to cook omelette)
SCRAMBLED EGGS WITH GRILLED TOMATO & SAUTÉED FIELD MUSHROOMS			
Field mushrooms & grilled tomato	Scrambled eggs	Wholegrain sourdough toast	Extra virgin olive oil (to cook mushrooms)
BUCKWHEAT PANCAKES WITH BERRIES & YOGHURT			
Mixed berries	Greek-style yoghurt	Buckwheat pancakes	Extra virgin olive oil (to cook pancakes)

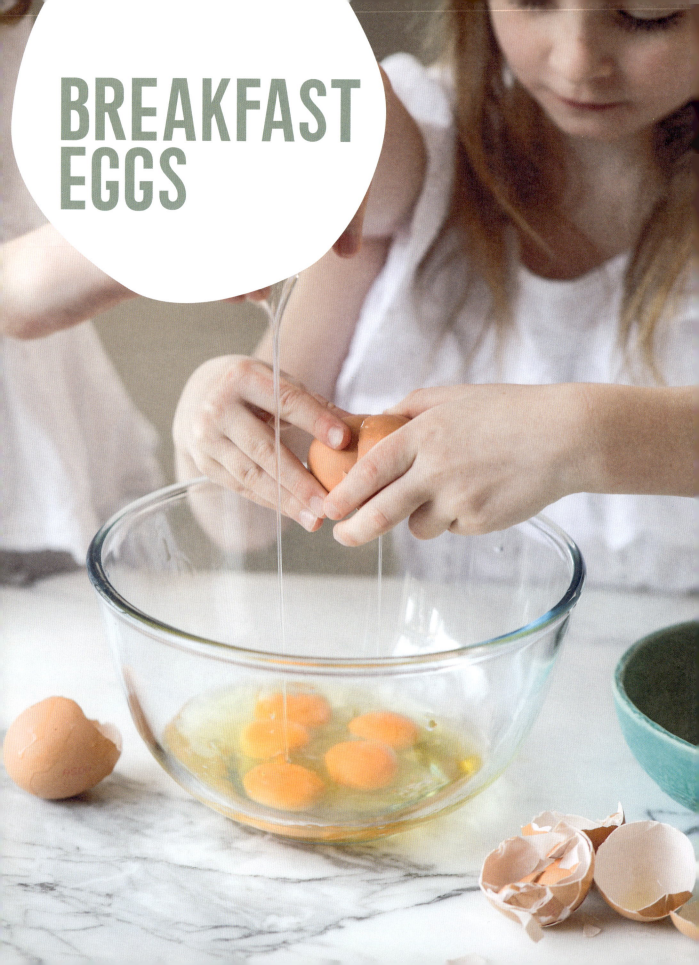

BREAKFAST EGGS

FRIED EGGS WITH HALOUMI AND GRATED VEGETABLES

PREP TIME: 5 MINUTES **COOK TIME: 5–10 MINUTES**

Getting a few vegies into breakfast is a great idea, helping you towards your 5 serves a day. This recipe is also perfect for using up any lone vegies lurking in the bottom of your fridge. Any root vegies will work, so feel free to replace the ones we've suggested – sweet potato, beetroot, turnip, swede and pumpkin are all good choices. And if you only have carrots, then make do with carrots!

SERVES 2

2 teaspoons extra virgin olive oil
½ carrot, grated
½ zucchini, grated
½ parsnip, grated
1 cup (150 g) sauerkraut
¼ cup coriander leaves
4 slices wholemeal sourdough
80 g haloumi cheese, sliced
2 large eggs

Heat the oil in a large frying pan over medium heat. Fry the grated vegetables for 2 minutes or until softened. Mix in the sauerkraut and coriander.

Move the vegetables to one side of the pan to keep warm.

Pop the sourdough bread into the toaster.

Meanwhile, add a little drizzle of extra virgin olive oil to the pan, if needed. Brown the haloumi on both sides and fry the eggs until just set.

Top the toasted sourdough with the grated vegetable and sauerkraut mixture, followed by the haloumi and eggs.

TIP

→ Drizzle a little sriracha chilli sauce over the top of each serving for a spicy kick.

nutrition per serve Energy **2030kJ** ‖ Protein **28g** ‖ Fat **19g** (Sat Fat 6g, Poly 3g, Mono 7g)
Carbohydrate **45g** ‖ Fibre **10g**

BOILED EGGS WITH MIDDLE EASTERN BREAKFAST PLATE

PREP TIME: 5 MINUTES   **COOK TIME: 10 MINUTES**

This is a great brekkie to whip up for the grown-ups, while boiling extra eggs to serve the kids. Many kids might also love this, or at least some of the ingredients. It's an easy recipe to adapt to suit everyone's tastes – scale up or down as needed.

SERVES 2

½ avocado, cut into wedges
2 tomatoes, sliced
100 g smoked trout or salmon
2 tablespoons labneh
1 teaspoon harissa
2 large eggs
4 slices wholegrain sourdough
1 teaspoon extra virgin olive oil
4 cups (200 g) baby spinach
½ lemon
1 teaspoon sesame seeds

Arrange the avocado, tomato, trout or salmon and labneh on two plates. Top the labneh with the harissa and set aside.

Bring a saucepan of water to the boil, reduce the heat to medium and gently add the eggs. Cook for 5 minutes for soft eggs or 7 minutes for hard-boiled eggs.

Meanwhile, pop the sourdough bread into the toaster.

Heat the oil in a frying pan over medium–low heat. Sauté the spinach until just wilted, then squeeze the lemon juice over the top and cook for 2 minutes or until the liquid has evaporated. Divide the spinach between the plates and sprinkle with the sesame seeds.

Peel the boiled eggs and cut in half. Add the sourdough to the plates, top with the eggs and serve immediately, sprinkled with some freshly ground black pepper.

TIP

→ To make labneh, put 300 g Greek-style yoghurt in a sieve lined with muslin or a clean tea towel and place over a deep bowl. Gather the edges of cloth together and secure with an elastic band, then strain the yoghurt overnight in the fridge. Discard the liquid and open the cloth to reveal the labneh.

nutrition per serve   Energy **2040kJ** ‖ Protein **31g** ‖ Fat **24g** (Sat Fat 6g, Poly 4g, Mono 11g)
Carbohydrate **31g** ‖ Fibre **10g**

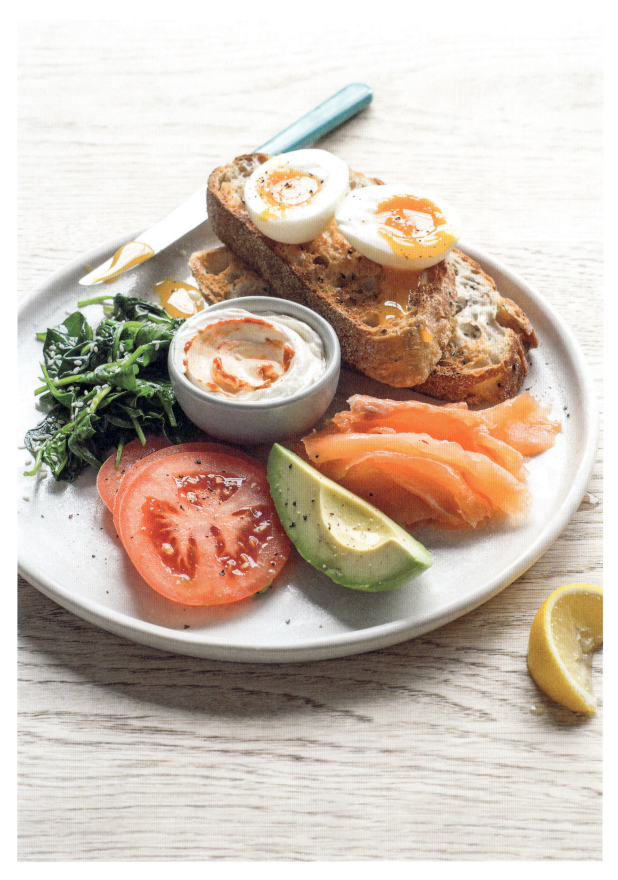

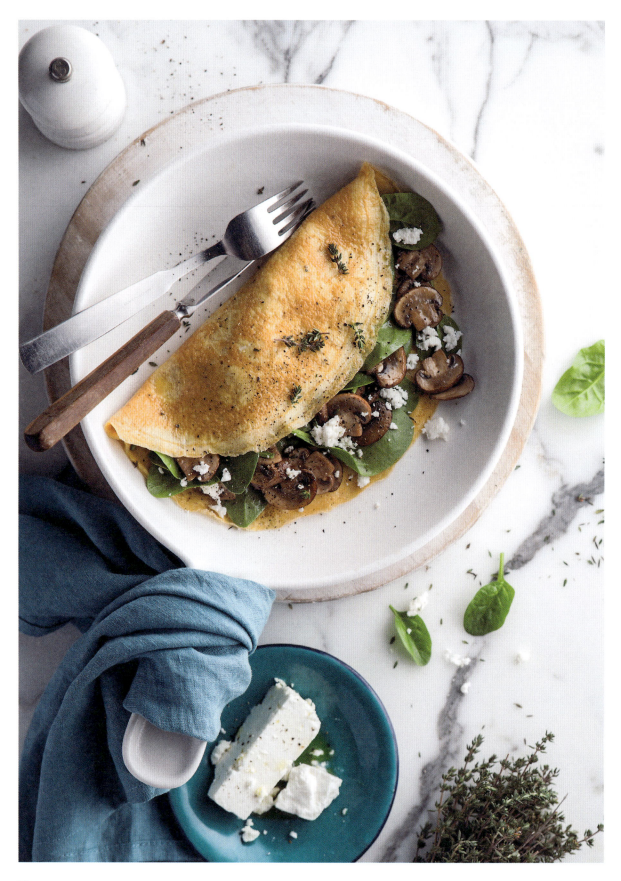

OMELETTE

PREP TIME: 5 MINUTES 🍳 **COOK TIME: 5–6 MINUTES**

SERVES 1

2–3 eggs
1 teaspoon extra virgin olive oil
Filling of your choice (see below)

Whisk the eggs in a bowl with 1 tablespoon water for each egg. Season with a grind of black pepper.

Heat a non-stick frying pan over medium heat and drizzle with the oil. Pour in the eggs and gently fold them over as the bottom sets (don't stir, or you'll end up with scrambled eggs!). Once about half the mixture has started to set, shake the pan to level it out and allow it to cook until almost set. Take care not to overcook the eggs – if your egg mixture is deep, you can put a lid on to help it cook through.

Add the filling ingredients to one half of the omelette and flip over the other half to enclose them. Continue cooking for 1–2 minutes to infuse the flavours and to melt the cheese, if using.

Slide the omelette onto a plate and enjoy immediately.

FILLING IDEAS

- → Goat's cheese, sautéed mushrooms, baby spinach and a pinch of thyme (pictured)
- → Cherry tomatoes, spring onion, baby spinach and grated cheddar cheese
- → Smoked or left-over cooked salmon, capers, sautéed or thinly sliced red onion, rocket and cream cheese
- → Left-over shredded chicken, ricotta or cottage cheese, tarragon, sautéed leek or onion, and tomato
- → Sautéed or marinated red capsicum, bean sprouts, prawns, fresh coriander and a drizzle of hoisin sauce
- → Or keep it simple with just a grating of parmesan cheese and serve with a salad to boost your plant food intake

nutrition per serve ┃ Energy **990kJ** ‖ Protein **19g** ‖ Fat **17g** (Sat Fat 4g, Poly 2g, Mono 9g)
Carbohydrate **<1g** ‖ Fibre **0g**
(3 eggs without filling)

POACHED EGGS WITH BAKED BEANS ON MUFFINS

PREP TIME: **5 MINUTES**   COOK TIME: **5 MINUTES**

This breakfast is a favourite with kids. It's so easy to whip up, and older kids can make it for themselves.

SERVES 2

White vinegar, for cooking
4 large eggs
220 g tin baked beans
2 wholemeal English muffins, split
20 g parmesan cheese flakes

Bring a saucepan of water to the boil. Add a splash of white vinegar to the water (this helps keep the egg white together). Carefully crack each egg into the boiling water, then cook for 3–4 minutes or until done to your liking.

Meanwhile, heat the baked beans in the microwave or in a small saucepan on the stovetop.

Toast the muffin halves.

Spoon the baked beans onto the muffin halves. Top each half with a poached egg and some parmesan and freshly ground black pepper. Serve immediately.

TIP

→ Add a handful of baby spinach leaves to the muffin halves before you add the baked beans – the heat from the beans will slightly wilt the spinach.

nutrition per serve   Energy **1750kJ** ‖ Protein **30g** ‖ Fat **13g** (Sat Fat 4g, Poly 2g, Mono 5g)
Carbohydrate **39g** ‖ Fibre **10g**

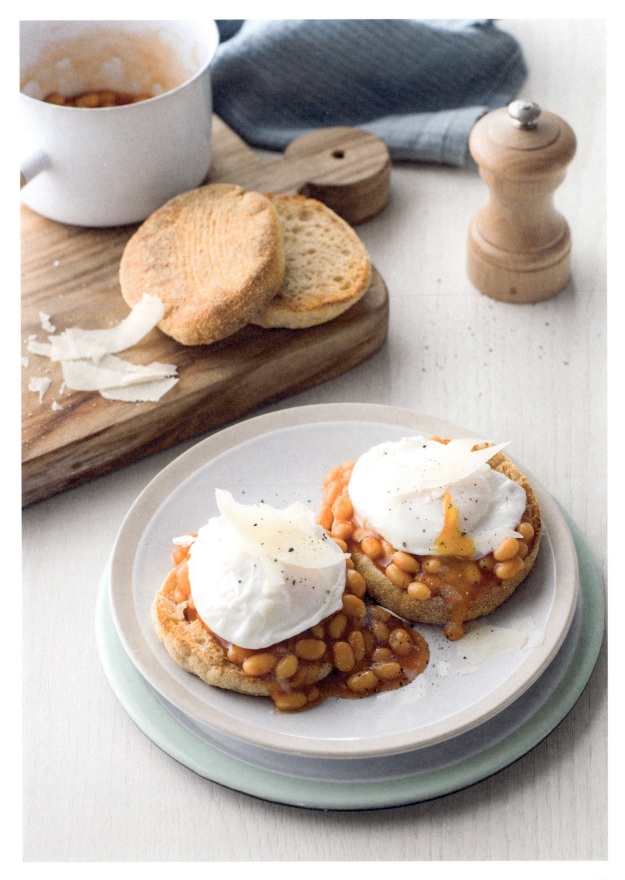

SHOULD WE BUY LOW-FAT DAIRY FOODS?

This is a very common question and it causes much confusion. Let's be clear: unless someone in the family has an allergy or an intolerance to dairy foods, both low- and full-fat dairy products are healthy options to include. They are valuable sources of good-quality protein and calcium, along with several other nutrients.

You certainly don't need to include dairy if you don't want to. However, if you choose to avoid dairy, be sure to include alternative food sources of calcium. A calcium-fortified plant milk is a good start. You'll also find calcium in tofu, edamame, leafy greens, teff, shellfish and dried figs, as well as in nuts and seeds, including tahini (sesame seed paste), almonds and chia seeds, and in the soft edible bones of sardines and tinned salmon.

If you do enjoy dairy, then whether you buy low- or full-fat products is really up to you. Children up to the age of two years should always have full-fat dairy foods because they need the extra energy and fat-soluble nutrients. From age two, there are some factors to consider.

→ Full-fat milk, cheese and yoghurt have, in recent research, been shown to be fairly neutral when it comes to the risk of heart disease. Despite being high in saturated fat, they do not raise your risk. It is perhaps the combination of the specific types of saturated fats present, along with the protein and calcium in these foods, that means the body deals with these differently than other sources of saturated fat. Nevertheless, they do contain considerably more kilojoules than their lower-fat counterparts, so portion size is important. If you have quite a lot of milk in your day – a few white coffees do add up – you might want to consider using low-fat milk to keep your kilojoules down.

Whether you chose full-fat, reduced-fat or low-fat dairy products, they're all full of beneficial nutrients.

→ Low-fat milk does not contain more sugar than full-fat milk. It's simply milk that has had the creamy layer removed. It has all the protein and calcium of regular milk.

→ Yoghurt is a stand-out beneficial food in nutritional studies. It may well be the fermentation process and probiotic bacteria present that exert benefits over fresh milk. It is incredibly versatile in both sweet and savoury dishes.

→ Cheese is also a fermented food and this may confer some benefits. And it's an excellent source of protein and calcium. Just watch your portion sizes as cheese is energy dense and easy to overeat.

→ Butter tends to raise blood cholesterol levels. It does not have the same nutritional benefits as whole dairy foods and it lacks both the protein and calcium. Butter does contain fat-soluble vitamins, but these can easily be obtained elsewhere. It's fine to use butter in small quantities, but since it lacks the impressive nutrition credentials of extra virgin olive oil, the latter is a better choice as an everyday fat.

→ Finally, what do you like? Personally, I don't like the creamy taste of full-fat milk, unless I actually want a creamy custard or sauce. I like the refreshing taste of skim milk and so do my kids, so that's what we buy. However, I always buy full-fat cheese as it tastes better! I would rather have the full flavour and truly enjoy it – plus, you can usually use less. When it comes to yoghurt, I use both full-fat and low-fat, depending on the purpose.

Take all of these factors into account and buy what's right for your family. When preparing the recipes in this book, we usually use reduced-fat milk and reduced-fat Greek-style yoghurt, and full-fat cheese, and this is what the nutrition analyses are based on. Substitute full-fat versions as you wish, but recognise that this will increase the kilojoules.

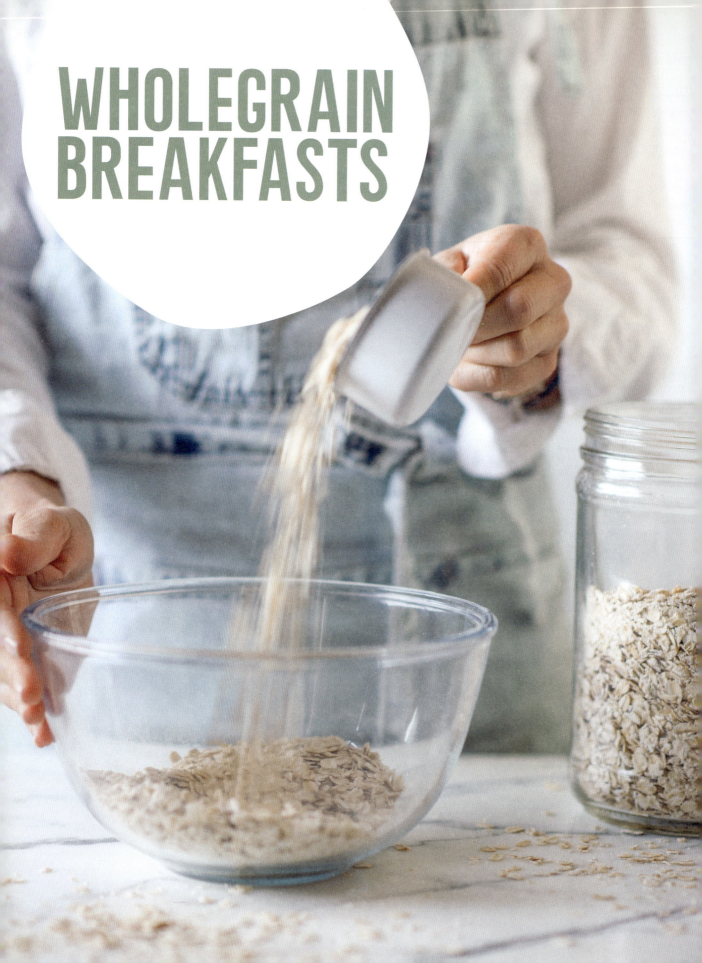

WHOLEGRAIN BREAKFASTS

BANANA BLUEBERRY BUCKWHEAT HOTCAKES

PREP TIME: **5 MINUTES** COOK TIME: **10 MINUTES**

It's hard to go wrong with hotcakes. You can whip up the batter the night before and leave it in the fridge to make them faster in the morning. Our version is gluten-free, but you can vary the flour. Use any wholegrain flour or boost the protein content with a legume flour such as lupin or besan (chickpea flour). You can also experiment with different nut meals.

SERVES 4

½ cup (65 g) buckwheat flour
½ cup (50 g) almond meal
2 teaspoons baking powder
¼ teaspoon mixed spice
2 large eggs, lightly whisked
⅓ cup (95 g) Greek-style yoghurt
1 teaspoon vanilla bean paste
2 bananas, mashed (about 230 g in total)
125 g fresh or frozen blueberries, plus extra to serve
2 tablespoons extra virgin olive oil

MAPLE YOGHURT
½ cup (130 g) Greek-style yoghurt
1 tablespoon pure maple syrup

To make the maple yoghurt, mix the yoghurt and maple syrup together in a small bowl. Set aside.

Mix the dry ingredients together in a bowl.

In a separate bowl, whisk the eggs, yoghurt, vanilla and mashed banana. Pour into the dry ingredients and stir to combine. Stir in the blueberries.

Heat half the oil in a frying pan over medium heat. Cook the hotcakes in batches, using ¼ cup of the batter for each one, for about 2 minutes on each side or until golden brown. Transfer to a plate with paper towel and keep warm while you cook the remaining batter to make 8 hotcakes in total, adding the remaining oil as needed.

To serve, place two hotcakes on each plate and top with a dollop of maple yoghurt and some extra blueberries.

TIP

→ Be sure to buy pure maple syrup and not maple-flavoured syrup, which is glucose syrup with flavourings added.

nutrition per serve Energy **1630kJ** ‖ Protein **14g** ‖ Fat **20g** (Sat Fat 3g, Poly 3g, Mono 12g) Carbohydrate **35g** ‖ Fibre **6g**

COFFEE OATS

PREP TIME: **5 MINUTES** COOK TIME: **5–6 MINUTES**

Oats are a fabulously nutritious grain, providing plant protein, bags of fibre and an array of vitamins and minerals, along with unique antioxidants that play a protective role in the body. This is a brilliant wake-up breakfast for grown-ups. You can leave out the coffee if you're cooking for younger kids.

SERVES 2

1 cup (95 g) rolled oats
1 cup (250 ml) milk
4 medjool dates, pitted and
    roughly chopped
1 heaped teaspoon instant coffee
    (or 2 shots of espresso)
½ teaspoon ground cinnamon
½ teaspoon vanilla bean paste
2 tablespoons natural or
    Greek-style yoghurt
100 g blueberries, raspberries
    or strawberries
20 g raw almonds, roughly
    chopped
2 teaspoons sunflower seeds
2 teaspoons chia seeds

Add the rolled oats, milk and 1 cup (250 ml) water to a small saucepan. Stir in the dates, coffee, cinnamon and vanilla. Cook over medium heat, stirring occasionally, until the mixture has thickened to the desired consistency. This should take about 5–6 minutes.

Divide the oat mixture between two bowls and top with the yoghurt, berries, almonds and seeds. Serve immediately.

TIPS

→ Add some sliced banana for extra fibre.
→ Replace the berries with diced seasonal fruit, such as peach, plum, rhubarb, apple or pear.
→ Shredded coconut makes a lovely topping.
→ For a nut-free version, substitute pepitas (pumpkin seeds) for the almonds.
→ For a dairy-free version, use a plant-based milk and omit the yoghurt.

nutrition per serve | Energy **1670kJ** ‖ Protein **16g** ‖ Fat **14g** (Sat Fat 3g, Poly 4g, Mono 6g)
Carbohydrate **47g** ‖ Fibre **11g**

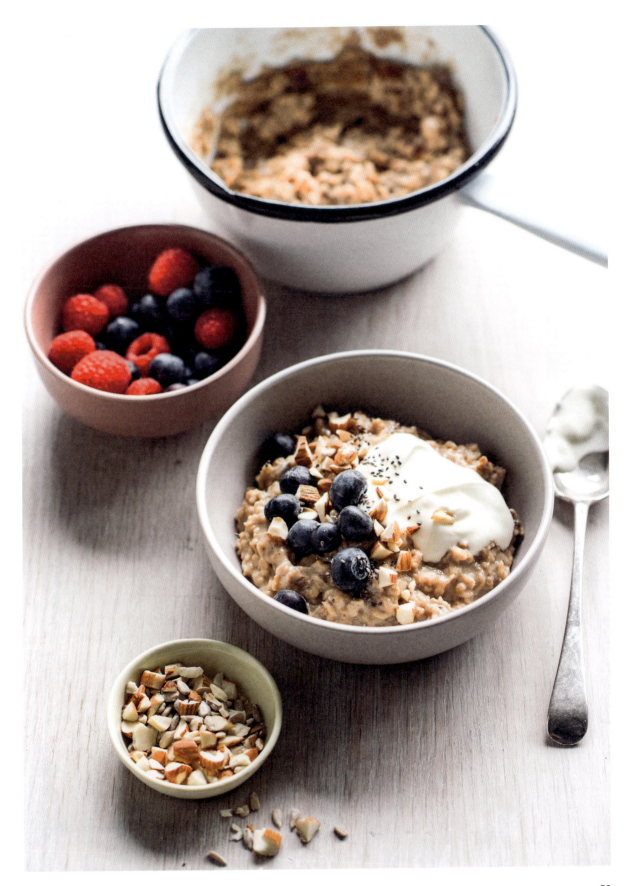

8 WAYS WITH TOAST

The most nutritious breads are those that are made with wholegrain flour. Look for the words 'wholegrain' or 'wholemeal' on the label. Multigrain bread usually contains mostly white flour with a few wholegrains added, but it is a step up from regular white bread. If your kids will really only eat white bread, buy those that have added fibre and/or a low GI. Sourdough breads are an excellent choice and usually have a lower GI. It's also a terrific idea to mix up grain varieties – try rye, barley, oat or ancient grain varieties.

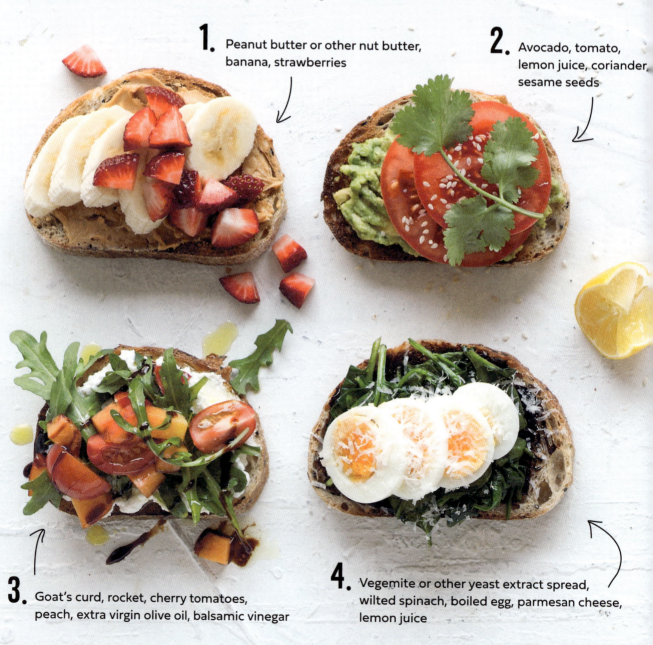

1. Peanut butter or other nut butter, banana, strawberries

2. Avocado, tomato, lemon juice, coriander, sesame seeds

3. Goat's curd, rocket, cherry tomatoes, peach, extra virgin olive oil, balsamic vinegar

4. Vegemite or other yeast extract spread, wilted spinach, boiled egg, parmesan cheese, lemon juice

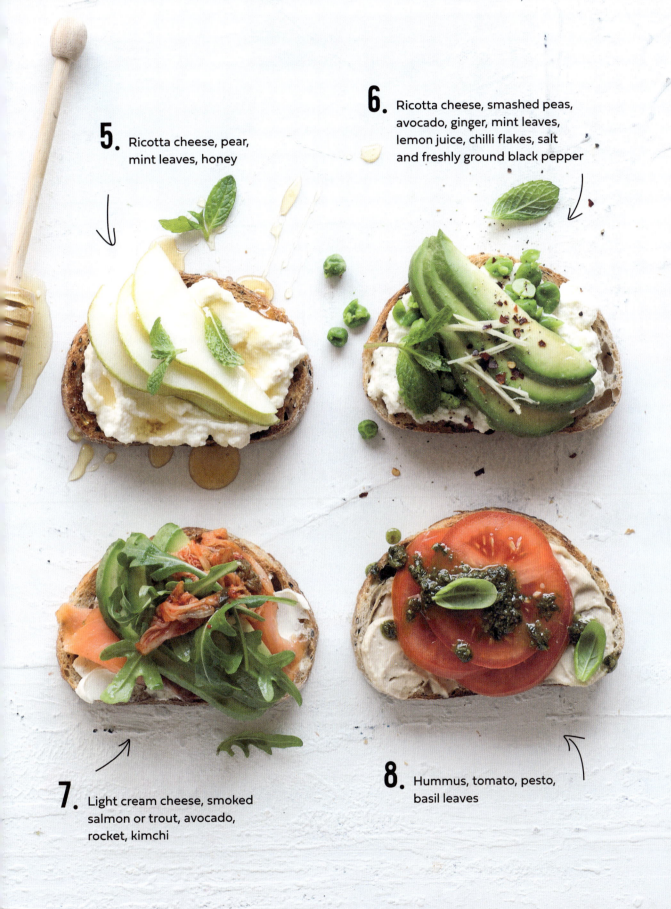

5. Ricotta cheese, pear, mint leaves, honey

6. Ricotta cheese, smashed peas, avocado, ginger, mint leaves, lemon juice, chilli flakes, salt and freshly ground black pepper

7. Light cream cheese, smoked salmon or trout, avocado, rocket, kimchi

8. Hummus, tomato, pesto, basil leaves

BEST-EVER LUNCHBOXES

The 5-step lunchbox planner

Packing lunchboxes doesn't have to be complicated – kids don't need endless variety, and it's enough to have a few options that they like and just rotate them. Use the Plate template (page 8) as your guide for packing lunchboxes. Think about how much your kids eat when they're at home for the day and remember that they typically have only two opportunities to eat at school – at morning recess and at lunch. Pack food accordingly and avoid giving them too much, or you'll just be frustrated at the waste. And if the lunchbox does come home with uneaten food, afternoon tea is sorted! Store the lunchbox inside an insulated bag, along with an ice pack, so the food stays fresh.

1. VEGIES & FRUIT

Here are some simple ideas to get vegies and fruit into lunchboxes:

→ Crunchy carrot and celery batons, a few baby cucumbers and/or cherry tomatoes alongside a sandwich or wrap
→ Raw vegie batons are also great popped into a container with a dip – try carrot, celery, capsicum and cucumber sticks with some hummus or guacamole
→ A sandwich or wrap with shredded lettuce, sliced tomato (remove the seeds so the bread doesn't go soggy), sliced cucumber, grated carrot, sliced or grated beetroot and roast capsicum pieces
→ Vegetable soup in a thermos container (blended soups are a great way to sneak in all sorts of vegies)
→ Whole fresh fruit (buy a banana container that prevents the fruit from getting bashed and bruised).

Products made with 100% fruit are not the same as whole fruit. Nutrients are lost in processing, and the body no longer has to break down the plant cell walls to access the nutrients and sugar to get the energy. These products are certainly a step above lollies, but consider them a healthier indulgence rather than an everyday food.

→ Sliced fruit or berries may be more likely to be eaten – a sliced apple or pear with a portion of cheese for recess, a container of mixed fresh berries, or a pot of Greek-style yoghurt topped with some passionfruit pulp or frozen berries (the berries will thaw by lunchtime, ready to stir through the yoghurt)

→ Tubs of fruit in fruit juice (not syrup) are convenient and easy to eat

→ Homemade muffins are terrific – make savoury muffins with vegies or sweet muffins with fruit

→ Smoothies in a thermos container – either blended vegies and fruit, or dairy or plant-based milk blended with berries or other fruit.

If your kids won't eat a beautifully prepared salad sandwich, don't despair. The most important thing is that kids eat mostly whole foods, with minimal junk foods. Encourage them to consume more vegies, but keep your eye on the big picture.

2. PROTEIN-RICH FOOD

Kids need protein at every meal to help regulate their appetite, provide amino acids for growth and development, and supply the micronutrients that accompany protein-rich foods. Here are some tips for how to include protein-rich foods in lunchboxes:

→ Cook extra meat at dinner, then slice it so it's ready in the fridge for sandwiches, wraps and salads

→ Poach a couple of chicken breasts, then slice and keep in the fridge

→ Ham is popular with kids, but it is high in salt and preservatives – try to limit ham to no more than twice a week, and buy ham sliced off the bone where possible, rather than highly processed ham

→ Cheese provides high-quality protein and is also an excellent source of calcium – add it to sandwiches and wraps, or add sticks of cheese with sliced apple or pear, or a couple of wholegrain crackers or oatcakes

→ Canned tuna and salmon provide high-quality protein and omega-3 fats that are essential for brain development – dress them with a little extra virgin olive oil and lemon, or whole-egg mayonnaise (smoked salmon and trout are high in salt, so watch the quantities)

→ Hard-boiled eggs can be packed whole as a snack or sliced and added to sandwiches, wraps or salads

→ Marinated tofu makes an excellent sandwich, wrap or sushi filling

→ Mix fresh (or frozen) fruit with natural yoghurt, or add a tub of yoghurt

→ Milk is an excellent drink that's rich in protein and calcium – freeze a small carton of milk and it will have defrosted and still be cold by lunchtime, or try making homemade flavoured milks or smoothies with dairy or plant-based milk, yoghurt and fruit, and store them in a thermos container.

Once you work out a few different options that your kids enjoy from each food category, mix and match them.

COMMERCIAL FRUIT YOGHURTS

Many parents are rightfully concerned about the amount of sugar in fruit yoghurts. However, bear in mind that the sugar listed on the nutrition panel includes the sugars that are naturally present in the milk and the fruit, as well as the added sugar. While the best option is to mix fruit with natural yoghurt so there is no added sugar, a tub of fruit yoghurt is still a healthy choice. It is low GI, rich in calcium and provides high-quality protein, and many brands are working to lower their added sugar levels. Steer clear of those with artificial sweeteners as these might have other negative consequences, such as impacting the gut microbiome.

3. SMART CARBS

There are lots of ways to include smart carbs in lunchboxes:
- → If you're making sandwiches, use wholegrain, low-GI breads and wraps
- → Beans, chickpeas and lentils contribute to the daily vegie servings and boost the protein – add them to soups or salads, or add beans to tuna mayonnaise sandwich fillings
- → Corn is great in sandwiches, soups and salads
- → Pasta (wholegrain is best but regular pasta is still low GI), brown rice, freekeh or quinoa can all be used in soups or salads
- → Homemade popcorn
- → Wholegrain muesli or cereal bars – make your own at home or use the Health Star Rating system to help you choose the healthiest ones
- → Use wholegrain flours to make muffins – try combining wholegrain wheat, kamut, spelt, quinoa, amaranth, lupin and besan (chickpea flour).

4. HEALTHY FATS

Below are some suggestions for adding healthy fats to lunchboxes. Remember that kids will also get some fat from meats, dairy and oily fish such as salmon and trout. And while most schools don't permit nuts, don't forget to give them to your kids at home – allergies excepted, of course.
- → Drizzle extra virgin olive oil over a pasta or rice salad
- → Hummus, mashed avocado, pesto and tahini are terrific in wraps and sandwiches.

5. WATER

Give your kids a refillable, stainless steel bottle of water. Be sure to empty and wash the bottle at the end of the day, and refill it with fresh water each morning. It's best not to send plastic bottles to school as the water is sitting in the bottle all day, and there is a risk of chemical leaching.

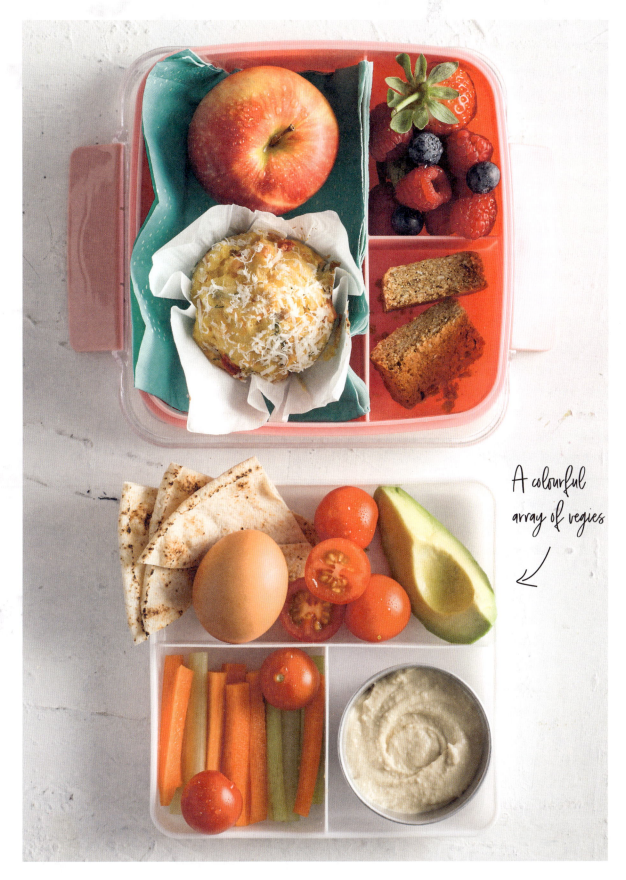

A colourful array of vegies

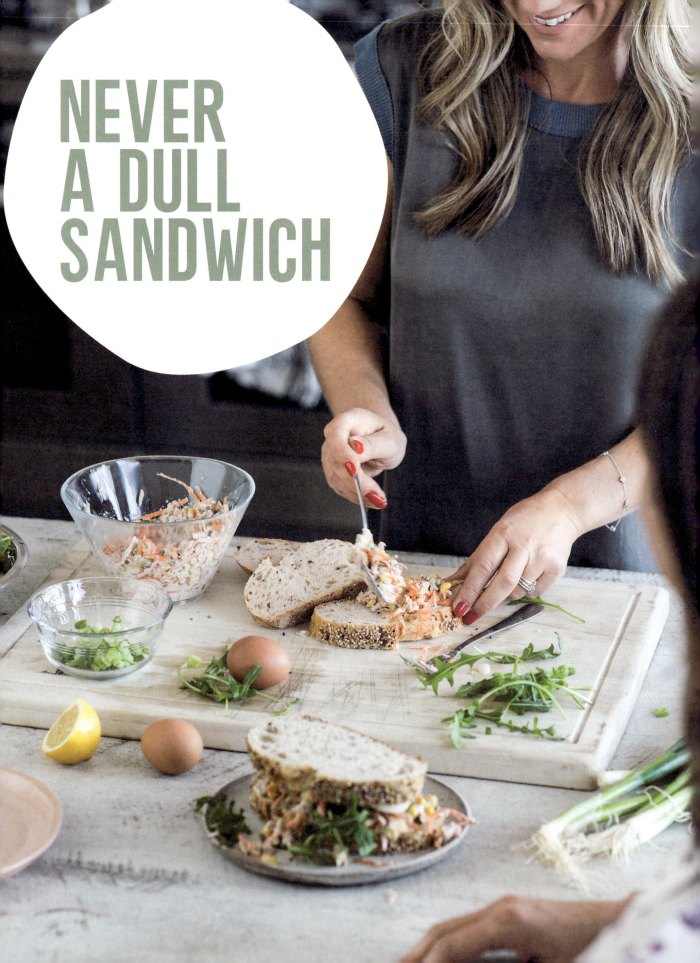

NEVER A DULL SANDWICH

THE STREAM: TUNA

PREP TIME: **5 MINUTES** COOK TIME: **NIL**

SERVES 2

Drain and mash a 185 g tin of tuna. Rinse and chop 1 teaspoon salted baby capers. Mix the tuna and capers with 40 g tinned corn kernels, 1 tablespoon finely chopped flat-leaf parsley, 1 thinly sliced spring onion, ⅓ cup (50 g) grated carrot and 1 teaspoon whole-egg mayonnaise. Season with freshly ground black pepper. Spread the mixture over 2 slices of wholegrain bread. Add 1 sliced boiled egg and 1 cup (45 g) baby rocket, and top with another 2 slices of wholegrain bread.

nutrition per serve

Energy **1310kJ** Protein **28g**
Fat **8g** (Sat Fat 2g, Poly 3g, Mono 2g)
Carbohydrate **29g** Fibre **7g**

TIPS

→ Try adding chopped tomato and olives to the tuna mixture.
→ Add sliced avocado to the sandwich before topping with the tuna mixture.
→ This mixture also works really well in a baked potato with a dollop of Greek-style yoghurt.

THE FARM: BEEF

PREP TIME: **5 MINUTES** COOK TIME: **NIL**

SERVES 2

Slice ½ small avocado and divide it between 2 slices of wholegrain bread. Top with 100 g sliced cooked lean beef, 1 thinly sliced tomato (seeds removed), 4 slices tinned beetroot and 1 cup (50 g) baby spinach or rocket. Spread 1 teaspoon dijon mustard over another 2 slices of wholegrain bread. Place on top of the rocket.

nutrition per serve

Energy **1290kJ** Protein **25g**
Fat **8g** (Sat Fat 2g, Poly 1g, Mono 4g)
Carbohydrate **30g** Fibre **8g**

TIPS

→ Try adding cheese, sauerkraut or kimchi.
→ Substitute the mustard for horseradish, relish or pesto.

THE VEGIE PATCH

PREP TIME: **5 MINUTES** COOK TIME: **5 MINUTES**

SERVES 2

Spread 2 tablespoons hummus over 2 slices of wholegrain bread. Top with ½ cup (125 g) diced roasted pumpkin, 1 cup (45 g) rocket or baby spinach, ½ cup (80 g) grated carrot, ½ cup (70 g) grated beetroot and 50 g pan-fried or grated raw haloumi cheese. Spread another 2 slices of wholegrain bread with 1 tablespoon Walnut, Basil and Spinach Pesto (page 171) and place on top of the haloumi.

nutrition per serve

Energy **1590kJ** ‖ Protein **18g**
Fat **15g** (Sat Fat 4g, Poly 3g, Mono 6g)
Carbohydrate **38g** ‖ Fibre **11g**

TIPS

→ Omit the walnut pesto for a nut-free sandwich. You could add tomato relish instead.
→ Try pesto with avocado, marinated or pickled vegetables, and tempeh or tofu.

THE COOP: CHICKEN

PREP TIME: **5 MINUTES** COOK TIME: **NIL**

SERVES 2

Combine 100 g shredded cooked chicken with 1 finely diced celery stalk and 1 cup (150 g) Asian Coleslaw (page 98). Spread the chicken mixture over 2 slices of wholegrain bread. Slice ½ small avocado and divide it between the sandwiches, then sprinkle with freshly ground black pepper and finish the sandwich with another 2 slices of wholegrain bread.

nutrition per serve

Energy **1390kJ** ‖ Protein **24g**
Fat **12g** (Sat Fat 2g, Poly <1g, Mono 6g)
Carbohydrate **29g** ‖ Fibre **7g**

TIP

→ If you're not avoiding nuts, add chopped walnuts or pine nuts, and some coriander leaves, mint leaves or sliced mango. You could also replace the avocado with pâté.

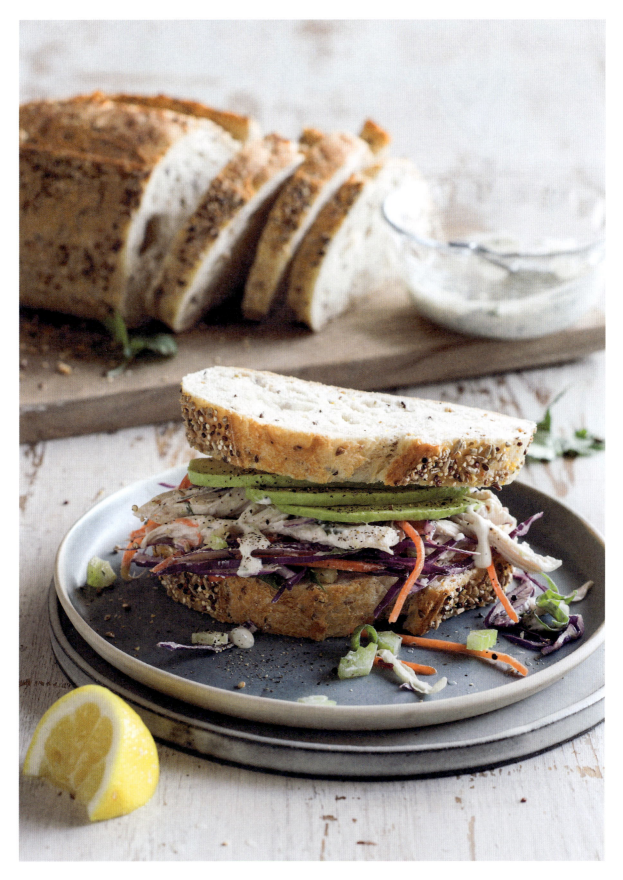

ENERGY FOOD

If kids are participating in a lot of sport, they'll need extra food to support their increased energy and nutrition needs. However, bear in mind that kids should be doing at least an hour of activity every day, and this won't require them to eat a lot more food. For adults as well as kids, it's a lot easier to consume kilojoules than it is to burn them off! If kids go overboard with extra snacks before or after sport, they risk gaining too much weight.

For the most part, if you stick to healthy food and drink options and encourage your kids to listen to their hunger cues, you'll get the balance right. Teach them about the importance of their food choices for giving them the energy for their chosen sport and don't use junk foods (including confectionery) as a treat for being active.

Think about the timing of food around sport – you wouldn't want to run around with a belly full of food, and your kids won't either. Giving them a big meal or snack right before sport will only result in them feeling sluggish or sick once exercising. If they're playing sport after school, pop an extra snack in their lunchbox to eat in the afternoon and, where possible, encourage them to eat it at least an hour before their activity.

If your kids are hungry on the way to sport, a banana or a small fruit smoothie are better choices than foods that take a while to digest. Liquids are emptied more quickly from the stomach and the carbohydrate from a drink or a banana will be absorbed fairly quickly and contribute to fuelling their muscles once they're exercising. Avoid giving them very high-fat foods or drinks, or those very high in fibre, as both will slow stomach emptying.

After exercise, kids need carbohydrates to restock the body's stores of glycogen in the liver and in the muscles. Plus, they'll need protein for muscle recovery, repair and growth. Don't overthink this – if you're heading home for a meal based on the Plate template (page 8), you already have it covered.

If your kids refuel after sport with smart carbs and protein-rich foods, and eat meals that are based on the Plate template (page 8), you'll have their energy and nutrient needs covered.

If a meal is some time away and the kids need a snack, here are some ideas that provide both smart carbs and protein:

→ Baked beans on toast or in a jaffle with cheese
→ A glass of milk with a muesli bar, healthy muffin or fruit loaf
→ Yoghurt with fruit and nuts
→ Nut butter on toast
→ A seafood sushi roll
→ A milk-based fruit smoothie (use dairy milk or a plant milk with a similar protein level, such as soy milk or oat milk).

When it comes to hydration, help kids get into the habit of drinking plain water. It's very unlikely that they'll need anything more than this – the meals and snacks that they eat before and after sport will replenish their glucose and electrolytes. Sports drinks will only serve to deliver extra kilojoules that kids don't need and get them accustomed to wanting sweet drinks... and they are dreadful for their teeth! The exception may be if your child is doing a long bout of exercise of over 90 minutes, or repeated exercise over a longer time frame, such as during a tournament. In these cases, watered-down fruit juice can be a good idea. It will give them some natural sugars to boost their blood glucose levels, while also hydrating them.

To make your own sports drinks:

→ If rehydration is most important (on a really hot day, or if your child sweats a lot), mix 1 part fruit juice to 3 parts water. This creates a drink that's absorbed faster than water alone (hypotonic).
→ If you want to provide energy and hydration, mix equal parts fruit juice and water. This creates a drink that will be absorbed in a similar way to water, but the added sugar will top up blood glucose levels when energy is flailing.

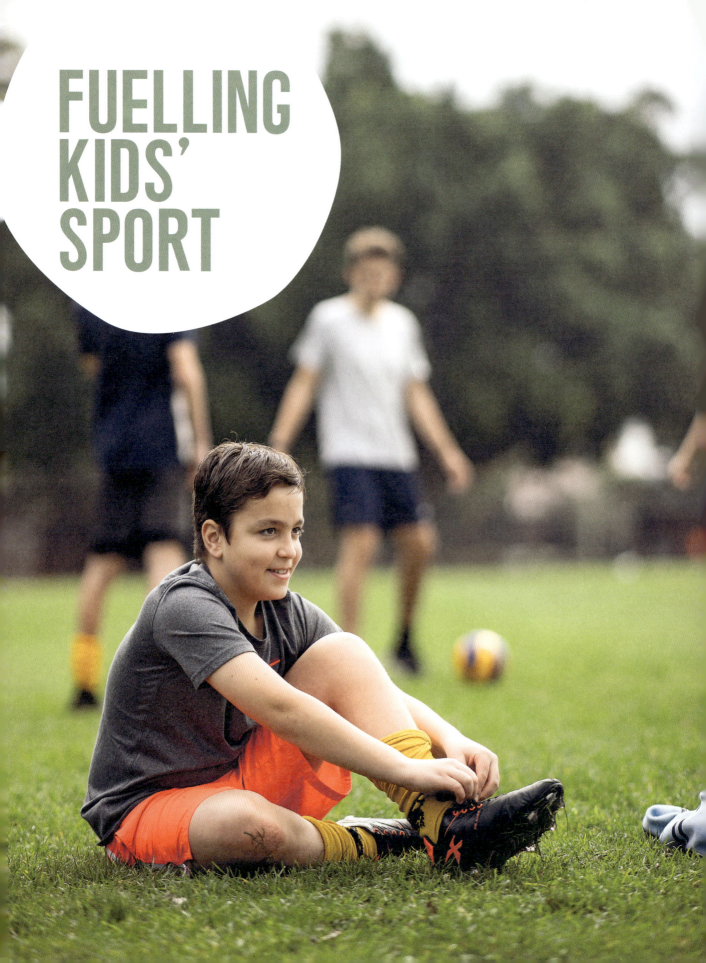

FUELLING KIDS' SPORT

COCOA BANANA PROTEIN SHAKE

PREP TIME: **5 MINUTES**   COOK TIME: **NIL**

Lots of teens start to get into protein shakes and sports bars. While there is a place for these foods, they are not a patch on whole foods. It's much better to steer clear of highly processed foods and powders. This natural, whole food protein shake contains 21 grams of protein and it comes with the complete nutrition package that's offered by real foods.

SERVES 1

1 cup (250 ml) milk
¼ cup (60 g) Greek-style yoghurt
1 banana
1 tablespoon almond butter
1 tablespoon chia seeds
1 tablespoon cocoa powder

Put all the ingredients into a blender and blitz until smooth. Pour into a glass or an insulated takeaway cup.

TIPS

→ Any nut butter can be used for a different flavour.
→ For a nut-free version, substitute tahini for the almond butter.
→ For a dairy-free version, omit the yoghurt and use oat or soy milk (most plant milks lack the protein of dairy milk – soy and oat have the highest protein content of all the plant milks).

nutrition per serve   Energy **1670kJ** ‖ Protein **21g** ‖ Fat **14g** (Sat Fat 4g, Poly 5g, Mono 5g)
Carbohydrate **41g** ‖ Fibre **11g**

BAKED MUESLI BARS

PREP TIME: **10 MINUTES, PLUS 5 MINUTES SOAKING** COOK TIME: **20 MINUTES**

You can, of course, buy muesli bars, but these homemade ones are so much tastier and well worth the effort. Make a batch on the weekend and they will last for a couple of weeks, if you can resist them for that long! For extra indulgence, drizzle a little melted dark chocolate over the top.

MAKES 18

⅔ cup (110 g) medjool dates, pitted
1 cup (95 g) rolled oats
½ cup (75 g) wholemeal plain flour
½ cup (45 g) desiccated coconut
¼ cup (35 g) pepitas (pumpkin seeds)
2 teaspoons baking powder
1 teaspoon ground cinnamon
Pinch of salt
140 g honey
180 g sunflower seed butter

Preheat the oven to 160°C. Line an 18 x 28 cm slice tin with baking paper.

Soak the dates in hot water for 5 minutes to soften.

Put the rolled oats, flour, coconut, pepitas, baking powder, cinnamon and salt in a food processor and process in short bursts until combined. Add the drained dates, one at a time, and process to distribute the dates throughout the mixture.

Add the honey and the sunflower seed butter and process until combined.

Spoon the mixture into the tin and firmly press it down with the back of the spoon. Bake for 15–20 minutes or until golden around the edges. Allow to cool in the tin before cutting the slice into bars. Store in a sealed container in a cool, dry place for up to 2 weeks.

TIPS

→ You can use any seed butter – try using sunflower, tahini or a combination seed butter. If you're not making the muesli bars for nut-free lunchboxes, you can use a nut butter instead.
→ For gluten-free muesli bars, substitute buckwheat flour for the wholemeal plain flour and use gluten-free baking powder.

nutrition per muesli bar Energy **700kJ** ‖ Protein **4g** ‖ Fat **8g** (Sat Fat 2g, Poly 1g, Mono 4g)
Carbohydrate **18g** ‖ Fibre **3g**

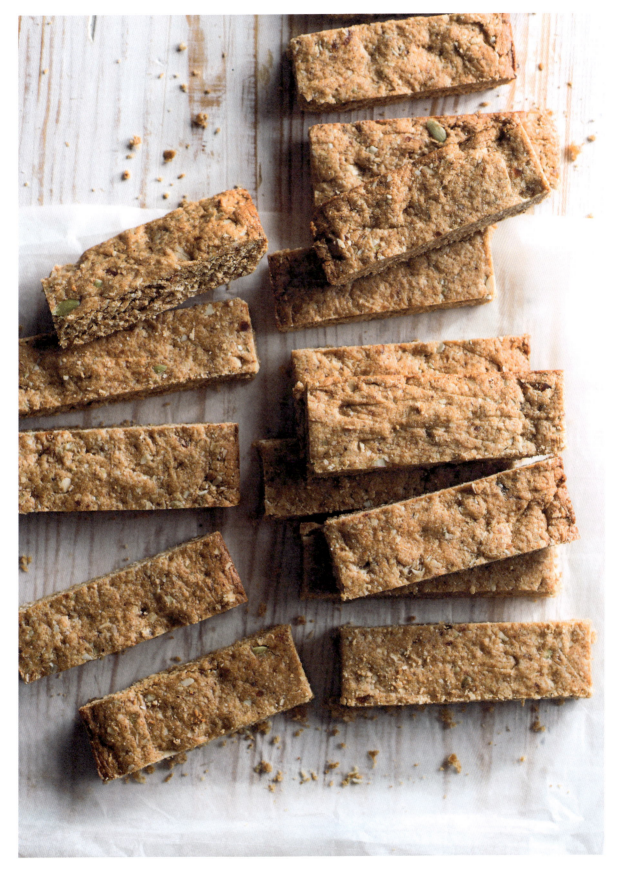

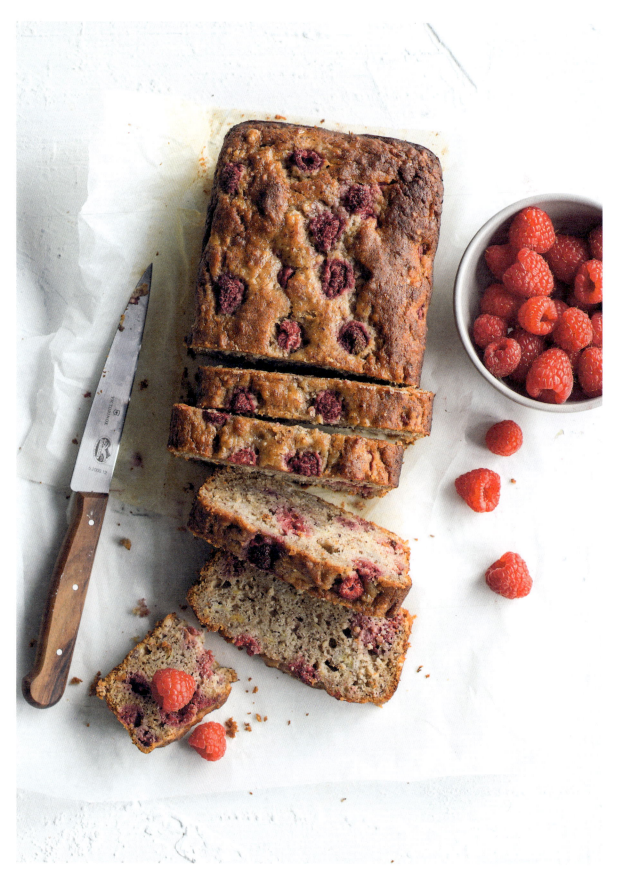

BANANA RASPBERRY NUT LOAF

PREP TIME: **10 MINUTES** 🍵 COOK TIME: **1 HOUR**

Commercial fruit loaves are usually made with white flour and refined oils, and are loaded with added sugar. Our super-tasty version uses buckwheat flour, nut meal and fabulously healthy extra virgin olive oil. You can slice and freeze it in individual portions and even thaw it directly in the toaster for a quick after-school snack. The grown-ups will also enjoy this loaf with an afternoon cup of tea.

SERVES 10

120 g buckwheat flour
100 g hazelnut meal
2 teaspoons baking powder
1 teaspoon mixed spice
3 ripe bananas, mashed
  (about 300 g in total)
⅓ cup (115 g) honey
2 large eggs, lightly whisked
¼ cup (60 ml) mild-flavoured
  extra virgin olive oil
1 cup (125 g) fresh or frozen
  raspberries

Preheat the oven to 180°C. Line a 10 x 20 cm loaf tin with baking paper, allowing the paper to extend over the sides.

Sift the flour, hazelnut meal, baking powder and mixed spice into a large mixing bowl.

Combined the mashed bananas with the honey, eggs and oil. Stir into the dry ingredients until just combined.

Reserve about 12 raspberries for decoration. Gently stir the remaining raspberries through the batter.

Spoon the batter into the tin, then top with the reserved raspberries. Bake for about 50–60 minutes or until the loaf is cooked through when tested with a skewer. If the skewer comes out sticky, bake the loaf for a further 5–10 minutes. Cool in the tin for 10 minutes before turning out onto a wire rack to cool. Store in the fridge for up to 5 days.

TIPS

→ Use a gluten-free baking powder for a gluten-free loaf.
→ You can replace the hazelnut meal with any other nut meal.
→ For a chocolate version, add 1 tablespoon dark chocolate chips along with the raspberries.

nutrition per serve   Energy **1010kJ** ‖ Protein **6g** ‖ Fat **13g** (Sat Fat 1g, Poly 1g, Mono 9g)
Carbohydrate **24g** ‖ Fibre **3g**

VEGIE RICOTTA MUFFINS

PREP TIME: 10 MINUTES 🍳 **COOK TIME: 30 MINUTES**

Savoury muffins are a nifty way of sneaking in a few extra vegies. They are lovely cold in lunchboxes or as an after-school or after-sport snack. You can also freeze these, although once thawed they are best warmed in the oven or microwave.

MAKES 12

¼ cup (60 ml) extra virgin olive oil
½ red onion, finely diced
½ red capsicum, finely diced
1 cup (150 g) wholemeal plain flour
1 cup (120 g) besan (chickpea flour)
3 teaspoons baking powder
2 large eggs
½ cup (115 g) ricotta cheese
¼ cup (60 ml) milk
1 carrot, grated
1 small apple, grated
½ cup (100 g) drained tinned
   corn kernels
Handful of basil leaves, finely
   chopped
A few dill sprigs, finely chopped
20 g parmesan cheese, grated

Preheat the oven to 180°C. Line a 12-hole muffin tray with muffin cases or brush with extra virgin olive oil.

Heat 1 tablespoon of the oil in a small frying pan over medium heat. Sauté the onion and capsicum for a few minutes, stirring frequently, until softened. Remove from the heat and set aside.

Sift the flours and baking powder into a large bowl.

Whisk the eggs in a separate bowl, then whisk in the ricotta, milk and the remaining 2 tablespoons of oil. Add the carrot, apple, corn and herbs and mix well, then pour into the dry ingredients. Mix until just combined, taking care not to overmix or you will end up with tough, dry muffins.

Divide the batter among the muffin holes. Top with the parmesan and bake for 25 minutes or until the muffins are golden brown and cooked through when tested with a skewer. If the skewer comes out sticky, cook the muffins for another 5 minutes and test again.

Leave the muffins in the tin for 5 minutes before transferring them to a wire rack to cool completely.

nutrition per muffin Energy **720kJ** ‖ Protein **7g** ‖ Fat **8g** (Sat Fat 2g, Poly 1g, Mono 4g)
Carbohydrate **17g** ‖ Fibre **4g**

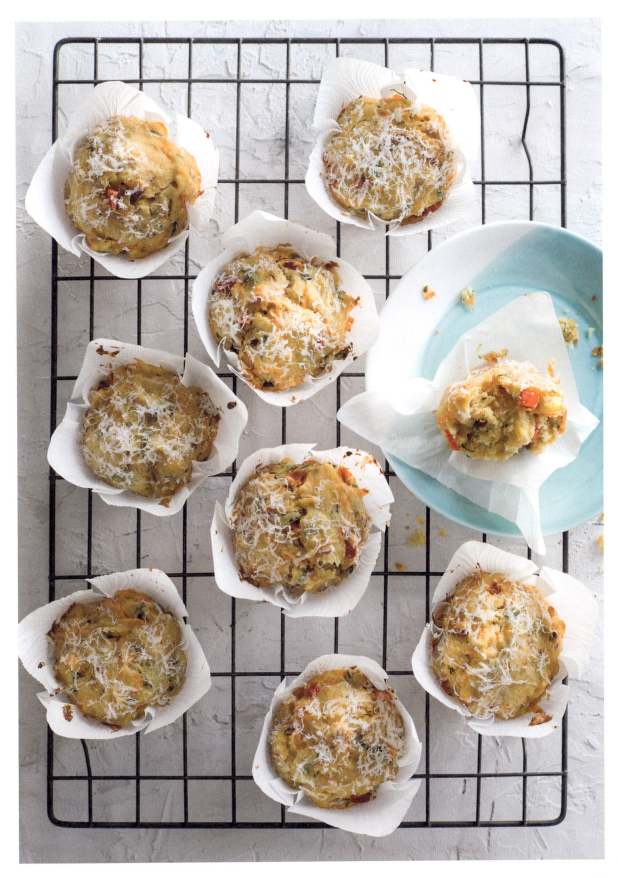

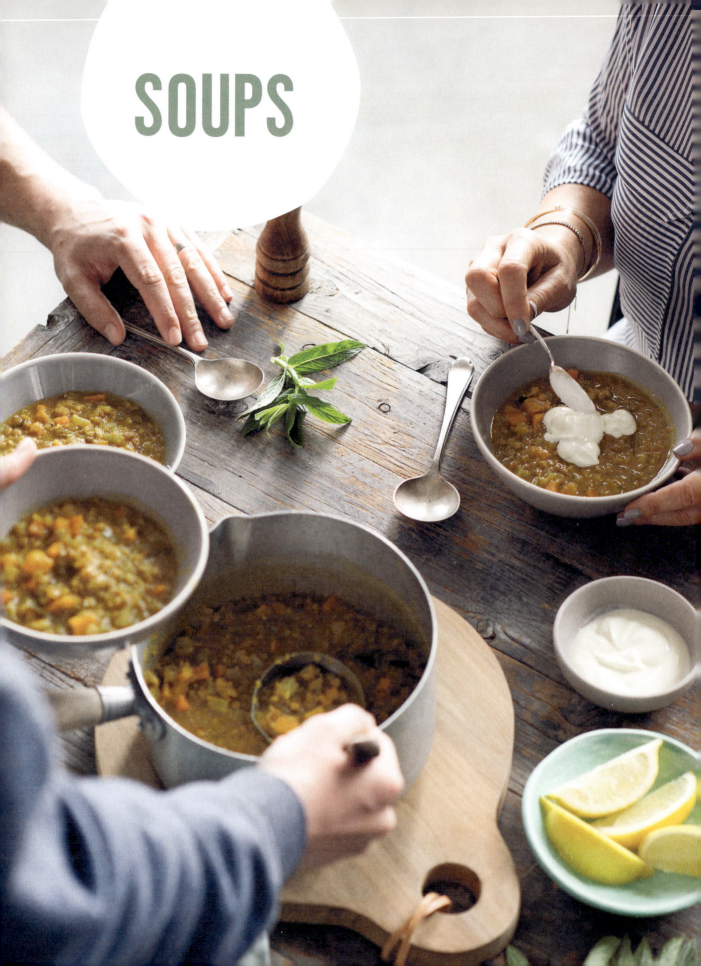

SOUPS

SUPER-QUICK ZUCCHINI SOUP

PREP TIME: **5 MINUTES** COOK TIME: **15 MINUTES**

This soup is terrific for helping you reach your target vegie serves for the day. The kilojoules are very low, so you have plenty of room to add a smart carb such as wholegrain bread, and boost the protein with some yoghurt or cheese. Alternatively, enjoy the soup as a first course and follow it with a main meal.

SERVES 4

1 tablespoon extra virgin olive oil
1 onion, roughly chopped
8 zucchini (about 800 g), roughly chopped
2 cups (500 ml) chicken or vegetable stock

Heat the oil in a saucepan over medium heat. Sauté the onion for 2–3 minutes or until translucent. Add the zucchini and cook until softened and slightly browned.

Pour in the stock and bring to the boil, then reduce the heat and simmer for 10 minutes or until the zucchini and onion are soft. Allow the soup to cool slightly before transferring it to a blender or food processor. Blitz until smooth, then season with salt and freshly ground black pepper.

TIPS

→ You can add 1–2 cups (50–100 g) of baby spinach when adding the stock, and a tablespoon of herbs such as mint, coriander or parsley for more flavour.
→ Sprinkle the soup with chopped nuts or seeds, such as pine nuts, sesame seeds or pepitas (pumpkin seeds). These add crunch as well as additional nutrients.
→ Serve the soup with a dollop of yoghurt and crusty wholegrain sourdough bread.

nutrition per serve   Energy **490kJ** ‖ Protein **4g** ‖ Fat **6g** (Sat Fat <1g, Poly <0.5g, Mono 3g)
Carbohydrate **9g** ‖ Fibre **5g**

TAMARIND LENTIL SOUP

PREP TIME: **20 MINUTES** COOK TIME: **45 MINUTES**

The tamarind and kaffir lime leaves add a fresh zing to this soup. The longer you simmer the soup, the deeper the flavour will be, and it tastes even better the next day. It's lovely topped with a dollop of natural yoghurt.

SERVES 6

1 tablespoon extra virgin olive oil

1 brown onion, finely chopped

1 garlic clove, crushed

10 g piece ginger, grated

1 lemongrass stem, pale part only, finely chopped

2 celery stalks, finely diced

1 carrot, finely diced

10 curry leaves

1 teaspoon ground turmeric

2 teaspoons ground coriander

2 teaspoons ground cumin

2 kaffir lime leaves, finely chopped

1 tablespoon flat-leaf parsley leaves, chopped

1½ tablespoons tamarind paste

1 cup (200 g) lentil soup mix, rinsed

2 cups (310 g) finely diced pumpkin

4 cups (1 litre) salt-reduced vegetable stock

2 tablespoons mint leaves

Heat the oil in a large saucepan over medium heat. Sauté the onion, garlic, ginger, lemongrass, celery and carrot until softened but not browned, about 2–3 minutes.

Add the curry leaves, ground spices, kaffir lime and parsley and cook, stirring, for 2 minutes or until fragrant. Stir in the tamarind paste.

Stir in the lentil soup mix and diced pumpkin, then pour in the stock and 2 cups (500 ml) water. Simmer the soup for at least 40 minutes.

Just before serving, season the soup with salt and freshly ground black pepper and top with the mint leaves.

TIPS

→ If the lemongrass is quite woody, blitz it in a food processor.

→ You can replace the kaffir lime leaves with the juice of 1 lime.

→ The soup is lovely topped with a dollop of natural or Greek-style yoghurt.

nutrition per serve Energy **860kJ** ‖ Protein **11g** ‖ Fat **5g** (Sat Fat <1g, Poly <1g, Mono 3g) Carbohydrate **28g** ‖ Fibre **7g**

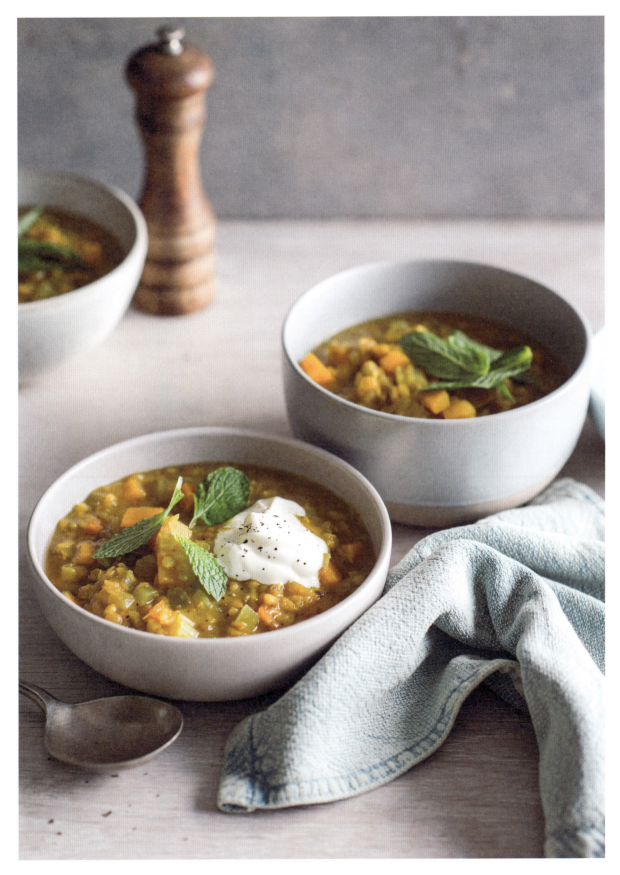

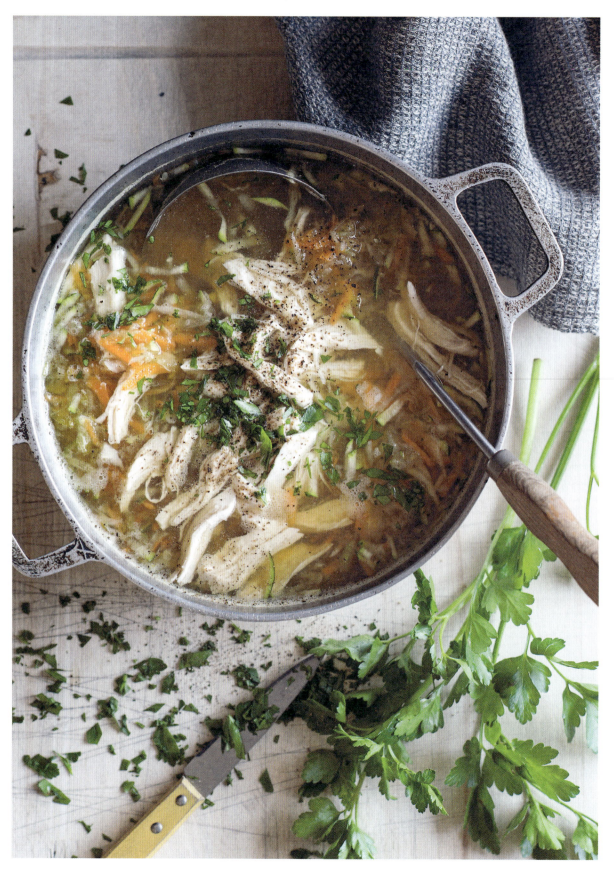

POP'S GRATED VEGETABLE AND CHICKEN SOUP

PREP TIME: **10 MINUTES** COOK TIME: **45 MINUTES**

Mel's pop used to whip up a batch of grated vegetable soup every week to keep the cold away. The secret to the beautiful sweet and savoury flavour in this soup is definitely the turnip. The other important ingredient is a good-quality chicken stock. Homemade stock is almost always better, but there are some good salt-reduced commercial varieties available.

SERVES 4

200 g skinless chicken breast fillet
2 carrots, peeled
1 turnip, peeled
2 celery stalks
1 zucchini
150 g butternut pumpkin, peeled
1 brown onion
8 cups (2 litres) salt-reduced
   chicken stock
⅓ cup flat-leaf parsley leaves,
   chopped

Put the chicken breast in a small saucepan and add enough water to cover the chicken. Bring to the boil over medium heat, then immediately reduce the heat and simmer for 10 minutes. Remove from the heat and leave the chicken to cool in the liquid while you prepare the vegetables.

Using the grating attachment on a food processor or a box grater, grate the carrots, turnip, celery, zucchini, pumpkin and onion. Transfer the grated vegetables to a large saucepan.

Shred the chicken and add it to the saucepan with the vegetables, then pour in the stock. Bring to the boil, then reduce the heat to a simmer and cook for 25–30 minutes or until the vegetables are soft and sweet.

Add the parsley and a good grinding of black pepper. Taste the soup and only add a little salt if necessary.

TIPS

→ Stir some baby spinach leaves through the soup just before serving so that they wilt slightly.
→ Add any other vegetables you have in the fridge.

nutrition per serve Energy **850kJ** ‖ Protein **26g** ‖ Fat **5g** (Sat Fat 1g, Poly <1g, Mono 2g)
Carbohydrate **10g** ‖ Fibre **6g**

PLANT-RICH EATING

Plant-rich eating is all the rage and with good reason. If there's one factor that unifies all dietary 'tribes', ways of eating and nutrition science research, it is the belief that eating lots of plant foods is a good idea for our health and the health of our planet.

Most experts around the world agree that there are two steps we need to take in order to minimise the environmental impact of farming and food production, and to be able to produce enough food to support our rapidly growing global population. We must lower our demand for animal foods (red meat in particular), and use more plant foods in their place.

What does plant-rich eating really look like? For some people, going all the way and embracing a vegan diet with no animal foods whatsoever is the right path. Others might choose to be vegetarian, and others might be pescatarian (they will eat seafood but not meat). For most of us, a more flexible approach to plant-rich eating is what works. This simply means eating more plant foods, perhaps choosing a night or two to opt for a vegan or vegetarian meal, and lowering our overall intake of meat and other animal foods.

Whatever path you choose in putting together the best diet for your family, we can all benefit from eating more plants.

TIPS FOR GETTING MORE PLANT FOOD INTO YOUR FAMILY'S DIET:

→ Try having at least one vegetarian dinner a week.

→ Have a handful of nuts a day as a snack in place of confectionery or highly processed bars and snacks that have a 'health halo' (such as most protein bars).

→ Expand the variety of vegies, fruit, wholegrains, legumes and nuts that you regularly eat. Diversity is king!

→ Grate or chop vegies to add to sauces, curries and casseroles – grated zucchini and finely chopped onion, garlic, carrot and capsicum work well in a bolognese sauce, while Asian greens, eggplant, okra and bean sprouts are fabulous in a curry.

→ Blend vegies with fruits to create different smoothies. Always blend rather than juice so that you maintain all of the nutrition in the plant.

→ Grate or chop fruit to add to porridge or baked goods – try grating apple or pear into porridge and add a teaspoon of cinnamon, and add chopped papaya or pineapple to a wholegrain muffin batter or fruit loaf.

→ Sprinkle chopped nuts or seeds over salads. They add a wonderful crunch and a burst of nutrition.

→ Be adventurous with wholegrains and look beyond white rice and wheat. Barley makes a wonderful nutty risotto, quinoa is perfect in salads, black rice is amazing with South American-style chicken, teff flour makes awesome pancakes, and oats can be used to make so much more than porridge!

→ Make a pot of vegie soup on the weekend and divide it into containers to use for lunch during the week. This is an ideal way to use up vegies neglected at the bottom of the fridge.

→ Make vegies delicious! While steamed crisp vegies on the side can be just right with a rich meat or fish dish, they can be a little boring. Drizzle vegies with extra virgin olive oil, sprinkle them with rosemary and garlic and roast in the oven. Or stir-fry vegies with ginger and chilli and top them with fresh herbs and sesame seeds. Make a ratatouille or stew with tomato and blend to make a rich vegie sauce to serve with pasta or meat.

→ Keep your pantry stocked with a mixture of different tinned beans, lentils and chickpeas and use them two to three times a week. Add them to soups or to meat dishes such as curries, casseroles and mince meals – you'll make the meat go further, while adding some plant protein, fibre and other nutrients. Toss them through salads. Mash them with extra virgin olive oil to serve with meat or fish. Or roast chickpeas with chilli and extra virgin olive oil to make a delicious snack.

→ Order an extra serve of vegies or salad when you're eating out. When ordering Thai food, for example, skip the white rice and order a serve of stir-fried vegies instead.

→ Experiment with tofu, tempeh and the new plant-based meat alternatives when eating out and for cooking at home.

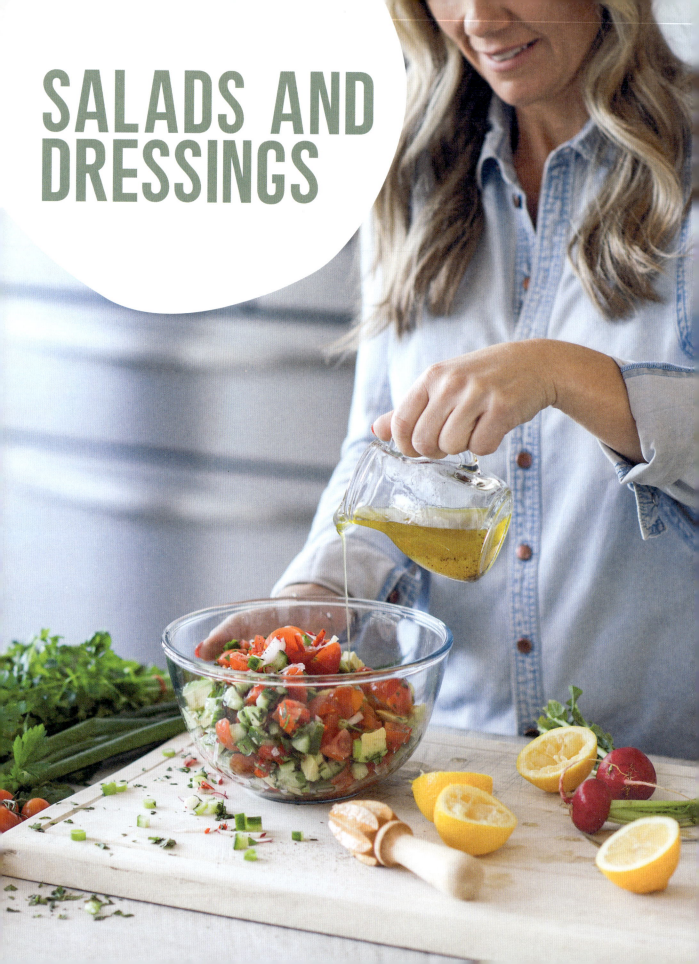

SALADS AND DRESSINGS

TOMATO SALSA SALAD

PREP TIME: **10 MINUTES, PLUS 20 MINUTES STANDING** COOK TIME: **NIL**

This versatile recipe is a salsa, a salad or a dressing! We use it in numerous ways, from a simple salad, to a dressing over grilled chicken, fish or haloumi, to a topping for nachos or tacos.

SERVES 6

2 cups (300 g) cherry tomatoes, quartered
1 Lebanese cucumber, finely diced
½ cup (80 g) finely diced red capsicum
½ cup (85 g) finely sliced radishes
½ avocado, finely diced (see tips)
2 spring onions, finely chopped
1 bird's eye chilli, finely chopped
1 heaped tablespoon flat-leaf parsley leaves, roughly chopped
1 tablespoon coriander leaves, roughly chopped
1 tablespoon mint leaves, thinly sliced
1 tablespoon extra virgin olive oil
1 tablespoon lemon juice
½ teaspoon salt
¼ teaspoon freshly ground black pepper

Combine the tomatoes, cucumber, capsicum, radishes, avocado, spring onion, chilli and herbs in a large bowl. Add the oil, lemon juice, salt and pepper and gently toss to combine.

Leave the salad to stand for at least 20 minutes before serving to allow the salt to draw out the juice from the tomatoes, creating a zingy dressing.

TIPS

→ You can leave out the avocado if you're serving the salad as a salsa with nachos, burritos or fajitas with a separate guacamole topping.
→ Add some tinned corn or black beans to the salad to make a salsa-style dip.

nutrition per serve   Energy **310kJ** ǁ Protein **1g** ǁ Fat **6g** (Sat Fat 1g, Poly <1g, Mono 4g)
Carbohydrate **3g** ǁ Fibre **2g**

SALMON, FENNEL, KALE AND BLACK RICE SALAD JAR

PREP TIME: **15 MINUTES**   COOK TIME: **NIL**

Jar salads make great portable lunches for the grown-ups. We've given quantities to throw together a salad for one, but you can scale up the ingredients to feed more people. The idea is to use left-over black rice from the previous night's dinner.

SERVES 1

2 tablespoons frozen peas
1 cup (50 g) finely chopped
    kale leaves
2 teaspoons extra virgin olive oil
⅓ cup (45 g) left-over cooked
    black rice
1 cup (50 g) baby spinach
1 tablespoon thinly sliced red onion
½ baby fennel bulb, thinly sliced
75 g left-over cooked salmon or
    hot-smoked salmon
¼ small avocado, diced
1 handful mint leaves
Squeeze of lemon juice
1 tablespoon peanuts,
    roughly chopped

Place the frozen peas in a small heatproof bowl, cover with boiling water and stand for 10 minutes. Drain the peas.

Meanwhile, put the chopped kale in a bowl and massage the leaves with 1 teaspoon of the oil for about 3–4 minutes or until softened. The leaves will turn from a matte sage colour to a dark green.

Put half the kale in a jar, followed by half the rice and half the spinach. Add the red onion and fennel, then add the remaining kale, rice and spinach. Add the flaked salmon, peas, avocado and mint.

Drizzle the remaining oil and the lemon juice over the salad, then sprinkle with the peanuts and put the lid on the jar.

TIPS

→ You can use a pre-cooked pouch or tub of microwavable wholegrain rice or grain mix instead of left-over black rice.
→ If you don't have any left-over cooked salmon, pan-fry a fresh salmon fillet in a drizzle of extra virgin olive oil. Alternatively, use a 95 g tin of salmon, tuna or mackerel in springwater.

nutrition per serve   Energy **1840kJ** ‖ Protein **27g** ‖ Fat **27g** (Sat Fat 5g, Poly 5g, Mono 16g)
Carbohydrate **18g** ‖ Fibre **9g**

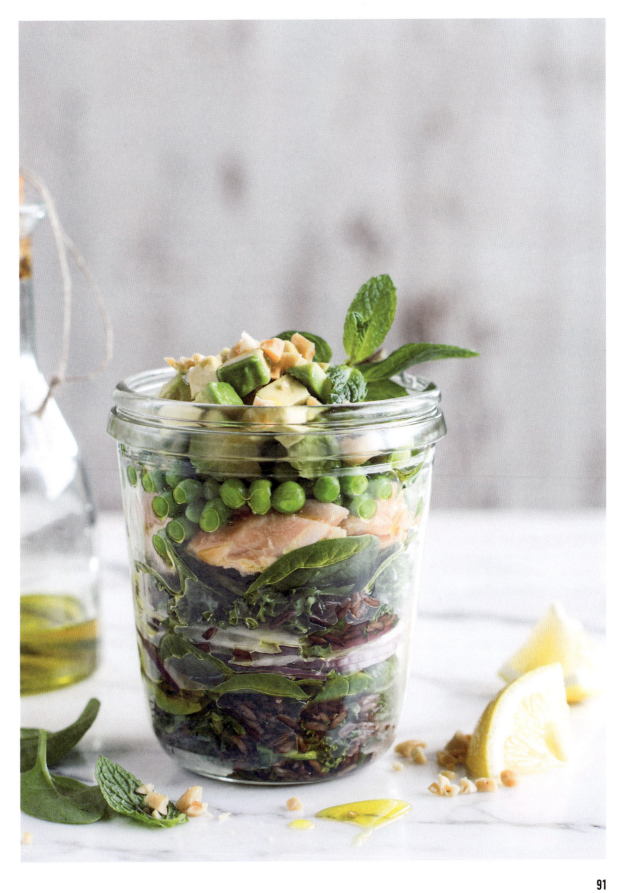

FREEKEH AND BLACK BEAN SALAD

PREP TIME: 20 MINUTES 👳 **COOK TIME: 15 MINUTES**

SERVES 6-8

1 cup (180 g) cracked grain freekeh
½ teaspoon salt
2½ cups (625 ml) boiling water
⅔ cup (80 g) hazelnuts
2 tablespoons sunflower seeds
2 tablespoons pepitas (pumpkin
    seeds)
400 g tin black beans, drained
    and rinsed
1 cup (200 g) tinned corn kernels
1 small red capsicum, finely diced
1 celery stalk, finely chopped
½ cup (80 g) diced red onion
3 spring onions, chopped
2 cups flat-leaf parsley leaves,
    finely chopped
¼ cup mint leaves, chopped
¼ cup coriander leaves, chopped
1 tablespoon salted baby capers,
    rinsed and chopped
Seeds of ½ pomegranate

POMEGRANATE DRESSING

⅓ cup (80 ml) extra virgin olive oil
1½ tablespoons pomegranate
    molasses
1 small garlic clove, crushed
Juice of 1 lemon
½ teaspoon honey or pure maple
    syrup

Put the freekeh in a large microwave-safe bowl along with the salt and boiling water. Cook on High for 14 minutes. Cover and stand for a further 10 minutes, then drain and set aside.

Meanwhile, lightly toast the hazelnuts, sunflower seeds and pepitas in a dry frying pan over medium heat for 2–3 minutes, shaking the pan occasionally. Allow to cool, then roughly chop.

Combine the freekeh, nuts and seeds with the remaining salad ingredients in a large bowl, reserving a few pomegranate seeds for garnishing.

Shake the dressing ingredients in a small screw-top jar until thoroughly combined. Taste and season with freshly ground black pepper and a little salt.

Stir the dressing through the salad, then scatter the reserved pomegranate seeds over the top.

TIPS

→ This salad is lovely topped with a dollop of tahini yoghurt. Mix ⅔ cup (190 g) Greek-style yoghurt, ⅓ cup (80 ml) lemon juice and 2 tablespoons tahini until smooth, adding a splash of water if it is a little thick.
→ Crumble feta or goat's cheese over the top of the salad to add a little salty bite.

nutrition per serve (8 serves) | Energy **1440kJ** ‖ Protein **11g** ‖ Fat **19g** (Sat Fat 2g, Poly 3g, Mono 12g)
Carbohydrate **28g** ‖ Fibre **11g**

HOISIN TOFU, BROCCOLI AND SUPER GRAINS SALAD

PREP TIME: **5 MINUTES**   COOK TIME: **5 MINUTES**

This is a truly satisfying salad to take to work or eat on the run. If you don't have any homemade hoisin dressing, you can substitute a store-bought Japanese sesame dressing. Delicious!

SERVES 1

80 g firm tofu, diced
1 tablespoon Hoisin Dressing
   (page 105)
1 cup (50 g) baby spinach
125 g microwavable wholegrain
   rice and grains mix
1 cup (60 g) broccoli florets
⅓ cup (35 g) sliced snow peas
½ cup (60 g) bean sprouts
1 tablespoon pickled ginger
2 teaspoons peanuts, chopped
½ cup coriander leaves
¼ cup mint leaves, torn
Wedge of lime

Toss the tofu in a bowl with the hoisin dressing to coat.

Put the spinach in the base of a lunch container or jar.

Heat the rice and grains mix according to the packet instructions, then allow to cool. Put the rice mix on top of the spinach.

Put the broccoli in a microwave-safe bowl with a splash of water and cook on High for 2 minutes. Refresh under cold water, then drain and place on top of the rice and grains mix.

Continue layering with the remaining ingredients, finishing with the marinated tofu. Serve with the lime wedge.

nutrition per serve   Energy **1820kJ** ‖ Protein **28g** ‖ Fat **13g** (Sat Fat 2g, Poly 5g, Mono 4g)
Carbohydrate **43g** ‖ Fibre **18g**

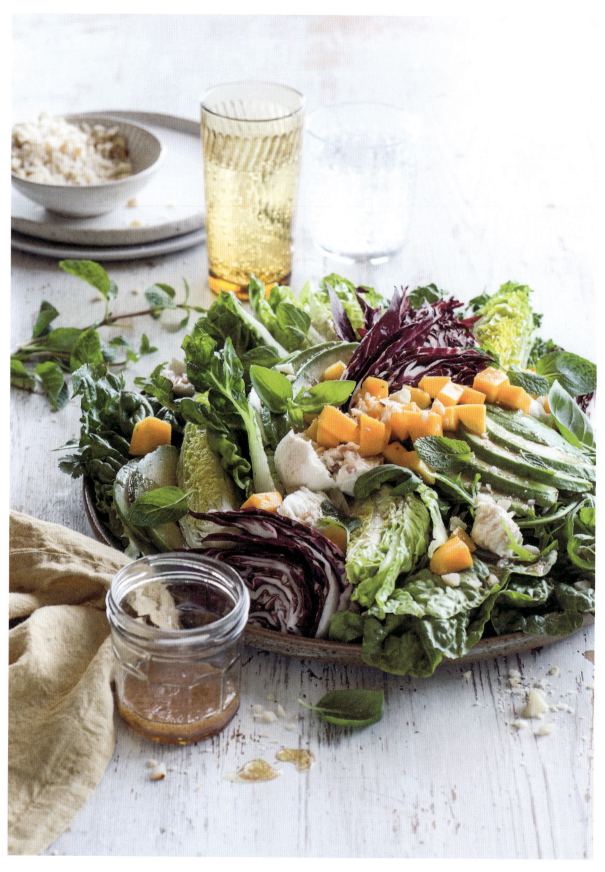

MANGO, AVOCADO, BOCCONCINI AND RADICCHIO SALAD

PREP TIME: 10 MINUTES **COOK TIME: 5 MINUTES**

This salad was created from random ingredients Mel had lying in her fridge. It's so easy, yet it looks fancy and sounds gourmet. It's a reminder to get creative with what you already have in the fridge or pantry.

SERVES 4

½ cup (60 g) macadamia nuts
2 baby cos lettuce, quartered
  lengthways
½ small radicchio, cut into wedges
2 cups (90 g) baby rocket
½ avocado, sliced
4 bocconcini cheese balls, torn
½ mango, diced
1 tablespoon small mint leaves
2 tablespoons small basil leaves

MUSTARD DRESSING
1½ tablespoons extra virgin olive oil
3 teaspoons red wine vinegar
1 teaspoon pure maple syrup
1 teaspoon dijon mustard

Toast the macadamia nuts in a dry frying pan over medium–low heat, shaking the pan occasionally. Watch carefully as the nuts can burn very quickly. Remove from the heat, transfer to a board and allow to cool. Roughly chop the cooled nuts.

Arrange the lettuce on a platter and top with the radicchio, rocket, avocado, bocconcini, mango and macadamia nuts. Sprinkle with the herbs.

To make the dressing, shake all the ingredients in a screw-top jar to combine. Season with a pinch of salt and freshly ground black pepper.

Pour the dressing over the salad just before serving.

TIPS

→ Try substituting any other type of nut for the macadamias.
→ This salad is delicious served with our Barbecued Chilli Prawns (page 155), or with a simple steak, chicken breast or fish fillet.

nutrition per serve Energy **1300kJ** ‖ Protein **8g** ‖ Fat **27g** (Sat Fat 6g, Poly 2g, Mono 17g)
Carbohydrate **8g** ‖ Fibre **4g**

BROCCOLINI, CHICKEN AND ROCKET SALAD

PREP TIME: 10 MINUTES **COOK TIME: 15 MINUTES**

Quinoa was once a trendy health food, but it is now more mainstream and available in most supermarkets. It is, admittedly, more expensive than rice, but nutritionally it ticks lots of boxes and another plus is that it cooks easily and quickly. You can always substitute brown rice, barley or bulgur if you prefer.

SERVES 1

¼ cup (50 g) quinoa, rinsed
½ cup (70 g) shredded cooked chicken
4 broccolini stalks, blanched and chopped
1 cup (45 g) rocket
¼ avocado, chopped
1 spring onion, thinly sliced
1 tablespoon mint leaves, finely chopped
1 teaspoon pepitas (pumpkin seeds)
1 teaspoon pine nuts, toasted
10 g parmesan cheese, shaved

LEMON YOGHURT DRESSING

1 tablespoon extra virgin olive oil
2 teaspoons lemon juice
¼ teaspoon dijon mustard
½ teaspoon Greek-style yoghurt
2 drops maple syrup

Put the quinoa in a small saucepan with ¾ cup (185 ml) water and bring to the boil. Reduce the heat, then cover and cook for 10–12 minutes or until the water has evaporated and the quinoa is light and fluffy. Turn off the heat and stand, covered, for 5 minutes.

To make the dressing, shake all the ingredients in a screw-top jar. Season with a pinch of salt and freshly ground black pepper.

Put the quinoa in a large bowl and add the chicken, broccolini, rocket, avocado, spring onion, mint, pepitas and pine nuts.

Transfer the salad to a serving plate or lunch container. Just before serving, drizzle with the dressing, to taste, and gently toss to combine, then sprinkle with the parmesan. Store any left-over dressing in the fridge for another salad.

TIPS

→ This salad works with any of the dressings from pages 104–105, including Blue Ranch Dressing (pictured).
→ Use left-over cooked chicken or a store-bought roast chicken. Or replace the chicken with smoked, hot-smoked or tinned salmon, and use goat's cheese or feta instead of parmesan.
→ You can serve the salad with a slice of wholegrain sourdough.

nutrition per serve   Energy **2430kJ** ‖ Protein **36g** ‖ Fat **33g** (Sat Fat 7g, Poly 6g, Mono 17g)
Carbohydrate **29g** ‖ Fibre **9g**

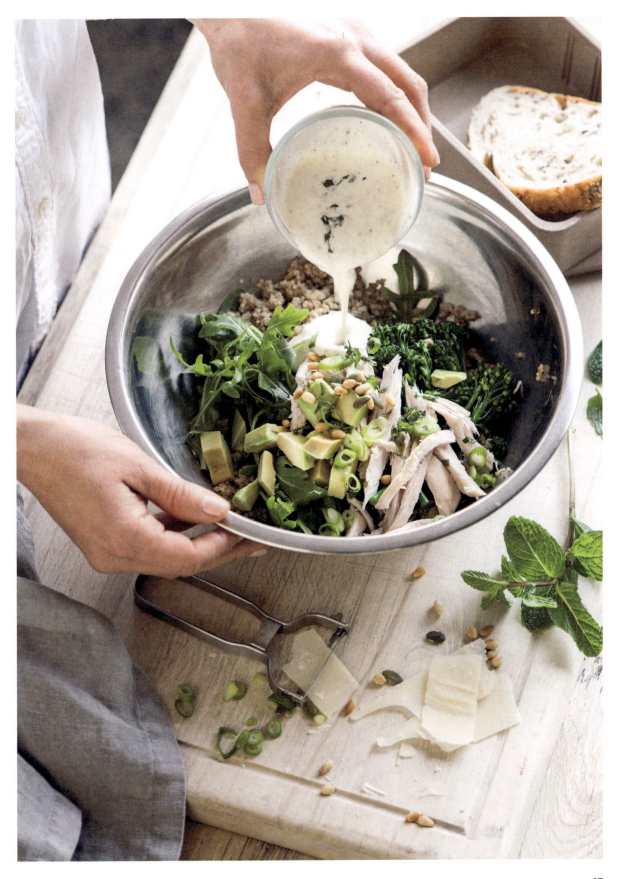

ASIAN COLESLAW

PREP TIME: **10 MINUTES** COOK TIME: **NIL**

There are so many ways to create a coleslaw – red, white or Chinese cabbage; vinaigrettes, Asian or sesame dressings; fresh herbs and aromatics such as dill, mint, coriander and chilli; and nuts and seeds have a place, too. You are only limited by your imagination. Anything works in a slaw... just go for it!

SERVES 4–6

2 cups (150 g) finely shredded white cabbage

2 cups (150 g) finely shredded red cabbage

1 cup (125 g) sliced green beans

3 spring onions, sliced

3 radishes, thinly sliced

½ cup (60 g) bean sprouts

⅓ cup coriander leaves, roughly chopped

2 tablespoons mint leaves, roughly chopped

⅓ cup (50 g) peanuts, toasted and roughly chopped

1 tablespoon white or black sesame seeds

100 ml sesame dressing (see tips)

Add the cabbage, beans, spring onion, radishes, bean sprouts, herbs, peanuts and sesame seeds to a large bowl.

Pour the dressing over the salad and toss to combine.

TIPS

→ You can buy sesame dressing from the supermarket or Asian grocer. Read the ingredients list to ensure you choose one with no nasties added!

→ Add some shredded cooked chicken or tinned fish to the coleslaw for a main-meal salad. Or serve it in wraps with your favourite meat or seafood.

nutrition per serve (4 serves) Energy **640kJ** ‖ Protein **6g** ‖ Fat **8g** (Sat Fat 1g, Poly 1g, Mono 5g)
Carbohydrate **12g** ‖ Fibre **5g**

CORN, FETA AND EGG SALAD

PREP TIME: 10 MINUTES 🍲 **COOK TIME: 10 MINUTES**

This is a wonderful salad to complement any barbecue. We particularly love it served with chicken or lamb skewers. Add the salad to a large bowl of leafy greens, and you have a feast ready for the whole family in next to no time.

SERVES 4

2 corn cobs, husks removed
2 spring onions, thinly sliced
2 tablespoons coriander leaves,
    roughly chopped
1 tablespoon mint leaves,
    roughly chopped
50 g feta cheese
½ avocado, diced
1 hard-boiled egg, chopped
1 tablespoon lime juice
1 tablespoon extra virgin olive oil
¼ teaspoon freshly ground
    black pepper
40 g grated parmesan cheese

Put the corn cobs in a saucepan of water and bring to the boil. Reduce the heat to a simmer and cook for 5–10 minutes or until the kernels are tender. Drain and refresh under cold water. Cut the kernels off the cob and place in a bowl.

Add the spring onion and herbs to the bowl and mix with the corn. Transfer to a serving dish and top with the crumbled feta, avocado and egg.

Drizzle the lime juice and oil over the salad, then season with the black pepper and sprinkle with the parmesan.

TIP

→ To save time, you can use tinned corn kernels instead of the fresh corn cobs.

nutrition per serve — Energy **1100kJ** ‖ Protein **11g** ‖ Fat **18g** (Sat Fat 6g, Poly 2g, Mono 8g)
Carbohydrate **12g** ‖ Fibre **6g**

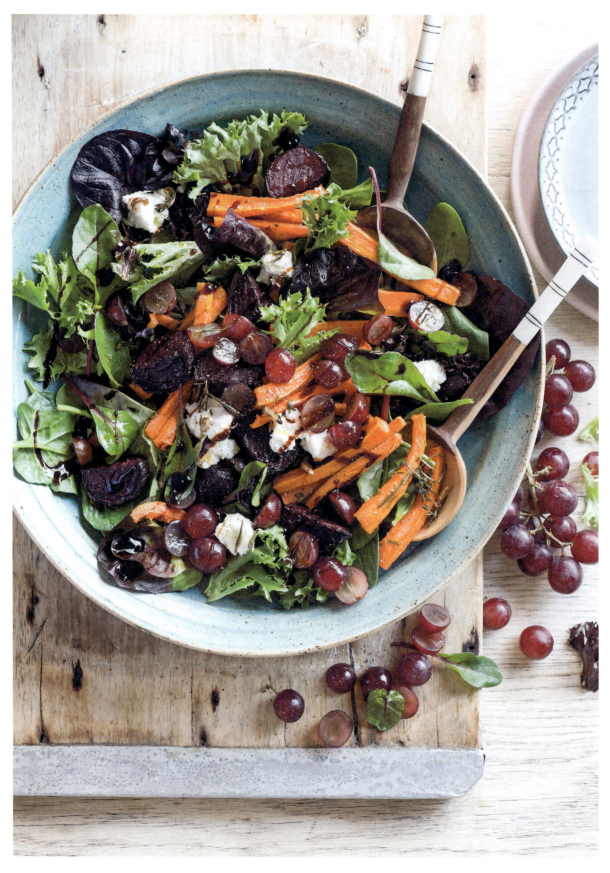

ROASTED BEETROOT AND CARROT SALAD WITH GRAPES AND GOAT'S CHEESE

PREP TIME: 10 MINUTES   **COOK TIME: 40 MINUTES**

This is a simple roasted vegetable salad that you can prepare ahead of time. Whenever we're roasting vegetables, we always roast extra with this salad in mind for the next night's dinner.

SERVES 4

- 2 garlic cloves, skin on
- 2 large beetroot, peeled and cut into 6 wedges
- 2 carrots, peeled and cut into batons
- 2 teaspoons rosemary leaves or ½ teaspoon dried rosemary
- 2 thyme sprigs
- 1 teaspoon thinly sliced ginger, skin on
- 2 tablespoons extra virgin olive oil
- 4 cups (200 g) mixed leafy greens, such as baby spinach and beetroot leaves
- ½ cup (90 g) small red grapes, halved
- ¼ cup (30 g) goat's curd
- 2 teaspoons balsamic vinegar

Preheat the oven to 180°C. Line a large baking tray with baking paper.

Bruise the garlic cloves with the side of a knife to release the flavour. Toss the beetroot, carrots, herbs, ginger and garlic in a bowl with 1 tablespoon of the oil. Sprinkle with salt and freshly ground black pepper.

Spread the vegetables over the baking tray in a single layer. Bake, turning once, for 30–40 minutes or until the beetroot and carrots are golden and cooked through. Allow to cool.

Toss the roasted vegetables with the salad leaves and grapes, then finish with dollops of goat's curd. Drizzle the salad with the remaining 1 tablespoon of oil and the balsamic vinegar.

TIP

→ You can substitute the grapes with fresh figs when in season, and replace the goat's curd with buffalo mozzarella or labneh.

nutrition per serve   Energy **980kJ** ‖ Protein **7g** ‖ Fat **14g** (Sat Fat 4g, Poly 1g, Mono 8g)
Carbohydrate **16g** ‖ Fibre **8g**

CHICKEN COBB SALAD WITH BLUE RANCH DRESSING

PREP TIME: **10 MINUTES** | COOK TIME: **2 MINUTES**

Corn is a wholegrain and counts towards your daily wholegrain target. It tends to be a favourite with kids and adults alike, so get creative with how you use it, although a simple steamed or barbecued corn cob is also delicious. Think ahead when you're cooking chicken on the barbecue – grill some extra along with some corn cobs and this salad will be a cinch to throw together for lunch the next day.

SERVES 1

40 g green beans, trimmed
1 cup (50 g) baby spinach
80 g cooked chicken breast, shredded
1 hard-boiled egg, halved
⅓ cup (65 g) tinned corn kernels
50 g cherry tomatoes, halved
60 g cucumber, cut into large chunks
¼ avocado, chopped
1 spring onion, thinly sliced
5 pitted black olives, halved
1 tablespoon dill, finely chopped
1 tablespoon coriander leaves, finely chopped
¼ teaspoon freshly ground black pepper
1 tablespoon Blue Ranch Dressing (page 105)

Put the beans in a microwave-safe bowl with a splash of water and cook on High for 1½ minutes. Drain and refresh under cold water.

Put the spinach, beans, chicken, egg, corn, tomatoes, cucumber, avocado, spring onion, olives and herbs in a large container and sprinkle with the pepper.

Pour the dressing into a small container to drizzle over the salad just before serving.

TIPS

→ If you aren't a blue cheese fan, this salad is equally delicious with a vinaigrette dressing.
→ Barbecued corn is beautiful in this salad – barbecue a cob of corn with a little extra virgin olive oil and a sprinkle of salt and freshly ground black pepper until tender and charred. Cut the kernels off the cob and store in a sealed container in the fridge to add to salads over a few days.

nutrition per serve   Energy **2140kJ** ‖ Protein **38g** ‖ Fat **31g** (Sat Fat 7g, Poly 4g, Mono 18g)
Carbohydrate **16g** ‖ Fibre **9g**

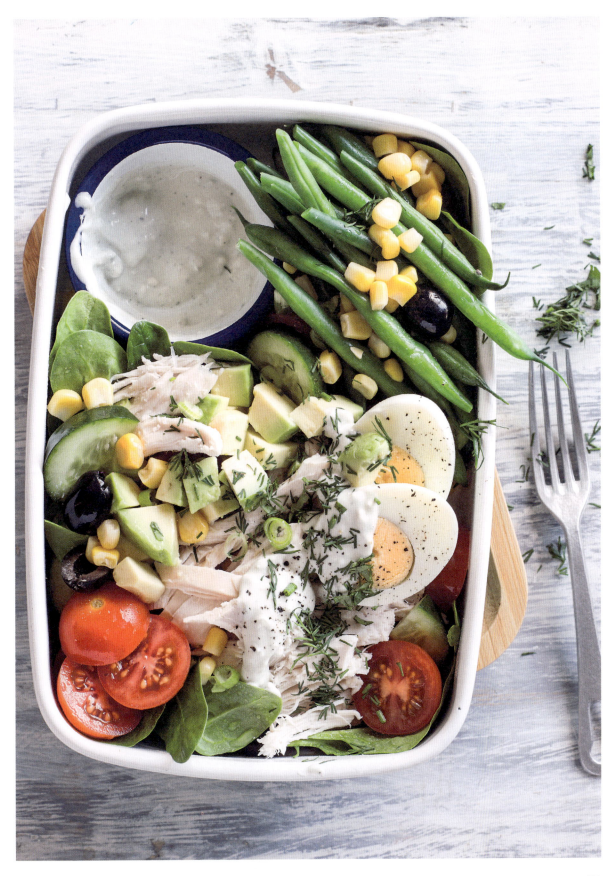

DRESSINGS

POMEGRANATE VINAIGRETTE

MAKES ABOUT ½ CUP (125 ML)

Shake ¼ cup (60 ml) extra virgin olive oil, 1 tablespoon lemon juice, 1 tablespoon pomegranate molasses, 1 teaspoon chopped mint, 1 tablespoon pomegranate seeds and ½ teaspoon freshly ground black pepper in a screw-top jar. Store in the fridge for up to a week. Bring to room temperature before serving.

nutrition per 1 tablespoon

Energy **380kJ** ∥ Protein **0g**
Fat **9g** (Sat Fat 1g, Poly 1g, Mono 7g)
Carbohydrate **2g** ∥ Fibre **0g**

SWEET ITALIAN VINAIGRETTE

MAKES ABOUT ½ CUP (125 ML)

Shake ¼ cup (60 ml) extra virgin olive oil, 1 tablespoon white wine or sherry vinegar, juice of ½ orange, 1 teaspoon honey and 1 teaspoon chopped oregano leaves or ½ teaspoon dried oregano in a screw-top jar. Store in the fridge for up to a week. Bring to room temperature before serving.

nutrition per 1 tablespoon

Energy **370kJ** ∥ Protein **0g**
Fat **9g** (Sat Fat 1g, Poly 1g, Mono 7g)
Carbohydrate **2g** ∥ Fibre **0g**

GREEN GODDESS DRESSING

MAKES ABOUT ½ CUP (125 ML)

Put ¼ cup (60 ml) extra virgin olive oil, 1 tablespoon lemon juice, 1 small strip lemon zest, ½ garlic clove, 1 large handful basil leaves, 2 tablespoons tarragon leaves, 2 tablespoons oregano leaves and 2 teaspoons water in a blender. Blend until smooth, transfer to a jar and store in the fridge for up to 4 days. Bring back to room temperature before serving.

nutrition per 1 tablespoon

Energy **360kJ** ∥ Protein **0g**
Fat **9g** (Sat Fat 1g, Poly 1g, Mono 7g)
Carbohydrate **0g** ∥ Fibre **1g**

TAHINI ORANGE DRESSING

MAKES ABOUT ½ CUP (125 ML)

Shake 1 tablespoon apple cider vinegar, 2 tablespoons orange juice, 2 tablespoons natural yoghurt and 1½ tablespoons tahini in a screw-top jar. Store in the fridge for up to 2 days.

nutrition per 1 tablespoon

Energy **160kJ** ‖ Protein **1g**
Fat **3g** (Sat Fat 0g, Poly 1g, Mono 1g)
Carbohydrate **1g** ‖ Fibre **1g**

BLUE RANCH DRESSING

MAKES ABOUT ½ CUP (125 ML)

Put ¼ cup (60 ml) extra virgin olive oil, 1 tablespoon lemon juice, 2 teaspoons yoghurt, 30 g blue cheese, 1 teaspoon chopped flat-leaf parsley, ½ teaspoon dill, ¼ teaspoon freshly ground black pepper, a pinch of cayenne pepper and a pinch of salt in a blender. Blend until smooth, transfer to a jar and store in the fridge for up to 2 days.

nutrition per 1 tablespoon

Energy **430kJ** ‖ Protein **1g**
Fat **11g** (Sat Fat 2g, Poly 1g, Mono 7g)
Carbohydrate **0g** ‖ Fibre **0g**

HOISIN DRESSING

MAKES ABOUT ½ CUP (125 ML)

Whisk ¼ cup (60 ml) hoisin sauce, 2 tablespoons extra virgin olive oil, 2 tablespoons lime juice, 1 teaspoon sesame oil, 1 teaspoon grated ginger and 1 teaspoon sesame seeds in a small bowl until smooth. Transfer to a jar and store in the fridge for up to 1 week.

TIP

→ You can use a store-bought hoisin sauce, but homemade sauce is so much tastier. Heat 1 teaspoon extra virgin olive oil in a small saucepan over low heat and cook 1 small crushed garlic clove and ½ teaspoon Chinese five spice until aromatic. Whisk in ¼ cup (60 ml) red miso paste, stir in 1 tablespoon brown rice vinegar and ¼ cup (60 ml) pure maple syrup and cook, stirring, for 1–2 minutes. Store in the fridge for up to 3 weeks.

nutrition per 1 tablespoon

Energy **370kJ** ‖ Protein **<1g**
Fat **8g** (Sat Fat 1g, Poly 1g, Mono 5g)
Carbohydrate **4g** ‖ Fibre **1g**

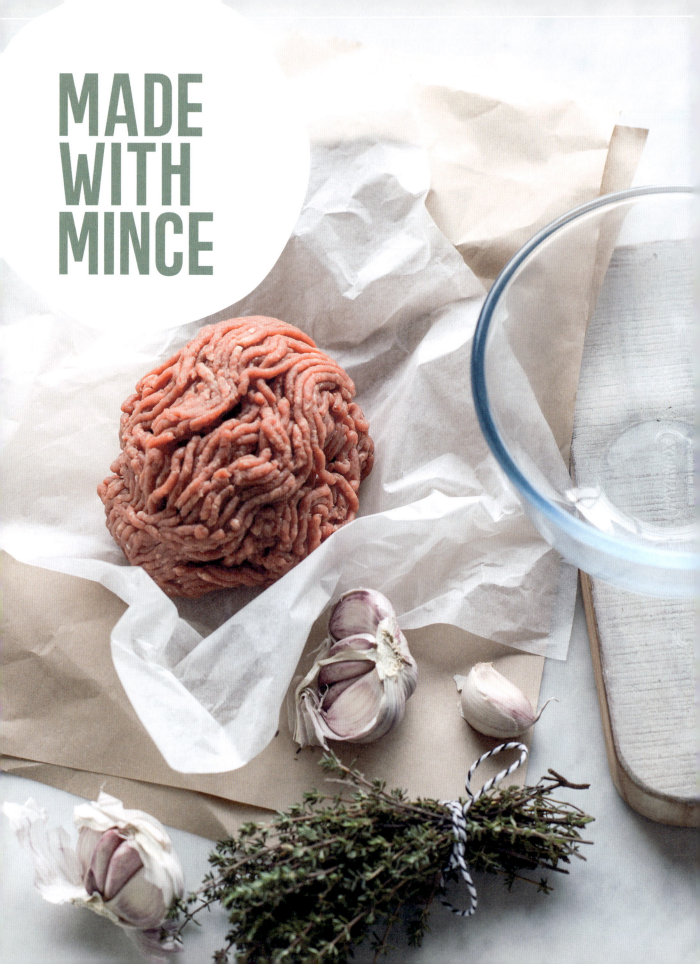

MADE WITH MINCE

CHILLI BLACK BEAN BOWL

PREP TIME: **15 MINUTES**   COOK TIME: **1¼ HOURS**

This hearty chilli is a versatile dish that can be served in different ways. We love it with black, brown, red or wild rice, topped with a spoonful of natural yoghurt, diced avocado, a little grated cheese and a few marinated jalapeño chillies, or as a taco filling.

SERVES 8

1 tablespoon extra virgin olive oil
1 red onion, diced
500 g lean turkey mince
500 g extra lean pork mince
2 celery stalks, diced
2 carrots, scrubbed and diced
1 red capsicum, diced
2 garlic cloves, finely chopped
    or crushed
1 tablespoon smoked paprika
1 teaspoon ground cumin
1 teaspoon ground coriander
1 long red or green chilli,
    finely diced
700 ml tomato passata
    (puréed tomatoes)
1 cup (250 ml) white wine or stock
1 teaspoon salt
420 g tin black beans, drained
    and rinsed
1 cup coriander leaves, roughly
    chopped
120 g baby spinach

Preheat the oven to 160°C.

Heat the oil in a large flameproof casserole dish over medium–high heat. Sauté the onion for 2–3 minutes or until softened. Add the turkey and pork and cook until browned, breaking up any clumps of meat. Add the celery, carrot, capsicum, garlic, spices and chilli. Cook, stirring, for 2–3 minutes. Stir in the tomato passata, wine or stock and salt.

Cover the casserole dish and transfer to the oven to cook for 1 hour. Halfway through the cooking time, stir in the black beans and check that there is enough liquid. Add a little water, if needed, then return the dish to the oven.

Just before serving, add the coriander and spinach to the chilli and stir until just wilted.

TIP

→ This recipe makes a large quantity of chilli. Freeze any leftovers in individual or family-sized portions.

nutrition per serve   Energy **1260kJ** ‖ Protein **31g** ‖ Fat **12g** (Sat Fat 3g, Poly 3g, Mono 5g)
Carbohydrate **13g** ‖ Fibre **8g**

FOUR-MINCE BOLOGNESE

PREP TIME: **15 MINUTES** COOK TIME: **2 ½ HOURS**

This recipe makes enough to freeze for several meals. We have snuck in loads of vegies and you can also add a tin of cannellini or borlotti beans.

MAKES 16 PORTIONS

2 tablespoons extra virgin olive oil
500 g extra lean beef mince
500 g extra lean pork mince
500 g extra lean lamb mince
500 g extra lean veal mince
2 brown onions, finely diced
4 celery stalks, finely diced
3 garlic cloves, crushed
1 large zucchini, grated
1 carrot, grated
1 cup (90 g) diced button
   mushrooms
1 cup flat-leaf parsley leaves,
   roughly chopped
1 cup (250 ml) white or red wine
140 g salt-reduced tomato paste
3–4 bay leaves
12 cups (3 litres) tomato passata
   (puréed tomatoes)

Preheat the oven to 180°C.

Heat the oil in a very large flameproof casserole dish. Add the beef, pork, lamb and veal and gently fry until browned, stirring to break up any large clumps.

Add the onion, celery, garlic, zucchini, carrot, mushrooms and parsley. Continue cooking for a few minutes until most of the liquid has evaporated. Stir in the wine, tomato paste, bay leaves and passata.

Cover the casserole dish and transfer to the oven to cook for 2 hours or until the sauce is rich in colour and flavour. Halfway through the cooking time, check that there is enough liquid. You may need to add up to 1 cup (250 ml) water to loosen the sauce. Return the dish to the oven. Season the cooked bolognese to taste.

TIPS

→ Leave the bolognese to cool before refrigerating overnight, then freeze it in family-sized portions. Heat it up and mix it with pasta shells in a thermos container for a great kids' lunch. Or use it to make nachos, tacos or burritos. It also makes a tasty jaffle filling with cheese.
→ If you have fussy eaters, sauté the vegetables separately, then purée and mix with the passata before adding to the meat.

nutrition per serve   Energy **1060kJ** ‖ Protein **31g** ‖ Fat **8g** (Sat Fat 2g, Poly 1g, Mono 4g)
Carbohydrate **11g** ‖ Fibre **3g**

SPICY MINCE WITH BEANS AND TOFU

PREP TIME: **15 MINUTES** COOK TIME: **45 MINUTES**

Don't be tempted to use firm tofu in this dish as it doesn't offer the same silky texture contrast of silken tofu, which is the beauty of this dish.

SERVES 4

1 cup (200 g) brown rice
300 g green beans, trimmed
1 tablespoon extra virgin olive oil
2 garlic cloves, crushed
2 teaspoons grated ginger
4 spring onions, chopped, white and green part separated
1 red or green chilli, chopped (optional)
500 g extra lean pork mince
2 teaspoons tamari or light soy sauce
1 tablespoon kecap manis (sweet soy sauce)
150 g silken tofu, finely diced
1 bunch broccolini
4 bok choy
¼ cup coriander leaves, roughly chopped
1 teaspoon sesame oil
1 teaspoon sesame seeds (optional)

Put the rice in a saucepan with 3 cups (750 ml) water. Bring to the boil, then reduce the heat, cover and simmer for 45 minutes or until the water has been absorbed and the rice is cooked. Turn off the heat and leave to stand without removing the lid for 5 minutes. Alternatively, cook the rice in a grain cooker.

While the rice is cooking, put the beans in a microwave-safe bowl with ½ cup (125 ml) water. Cover and cook on High for 1½ minutes. Alternatively, toss the beans in a wok over medium heat with a splash of water until just tender. Drain the beans, then plunge into ice-cold water. This stops the cooking process and helps to keep the bright green colour. Set aside.

Heat the oil in a large frying pan over medium heat. Gently fry the garlic, ginger, white part of the spring onions and the chilli, if using, until softened but not coloured. Add the pork and gently fry until browned. Add the beans and toss to combine. Stir in the tamari and kecap manis. Gently stir in the tofu and cook until heated through.

Put the broccolini and bok choy in a microwave-safe bowl with a splash of water and cook on High for 2 minutes. Alternatively, toss the vegetables in a wok over medium heat with a splash of water until just tender.

Transfer the pork mixture to a serving plate and sprinkle with the coriander and the green part of the spring onion. Drizzle with the sesame oil and finish with a sprinkle of sesame seeds, if using. Serve immediately with the brown rice, broccolini and bok choy.

nutrition per serve Energy **2170kJ** ‖ Protein **38g** ‖ Fat **15g** (Sat Fat 4g, Poly 3g, Mono 7g)
Carbohydrate **50g** ‖ Fibre **11g**

RICOTTA ZUCCHINI MEATBALLS IN TOMATO SAUCE

PREP TIME: 20 MINUTES COOK TIME: **45 MINUTES**

This recipe makes enough meatballs for two meals for a family of four, so you can serve half now and freeze the rest for another meal with a fresh batch of polenta. Admittedly, if you have hungry teenagers they may devour it in one meal!

SERVES 8

500 g extra lean beef mince
500 g extra lean pork mince
1 large zucchini, grated
1½ cups (150 g) finely diced
   mushrooms
1 large onion, finely chopped
1 garlic clove, crushed
⅓ cup flat-leaf parsley leaves,
   finely chopped
2 tablespoons salted capers,
   rinsed and chopped
½ cup (115 g) ricotta cheese
2 large eggs
½ teaspoon ground black pepper
1 tablespoon extra virgin olive oil
700 ml jar tomato passata
   (puréed tomatoes)
Basil leaves, to serve

SOFT POLENTA (SERVES 4)

1 teaspoon salt
1 cup (190 g) polenta
½ cup (40 g) grated parmesan
   cheese
1 tablespoon extra virgin olive oil

Add the beef, pork, zucchini, mushrooms, onion, garlic, parsley, capers, ricotta, eggs and pepper to a large bowl. Mix with your hands until well combined. Roll the mixture into balls about the size of a golf ball.

Preheat the oven to 180°C.

Heat the oil in a large ovenproof frying pan over medium heat. Gently fry the meatballs in several batches until browned all over, adding a little more oil to cook each batch if necessary.

Return all of the meatballs to the pan and pour in the tomato passata. Half-fill the passata jar with water and shake to loosen the remaining tomato, then pour into the pan. Cover the pan and transfer to the oven. Bake for 30–35 minutes or until the sauce is rich in colour.

After the meatballs have been cooking for 15 minutes, cook the polenta. Combine 4 cups (1 litre) water and the salt in a saucepan and bring to the boil. Slowly pour in the polenta while whisking to ensure there are no lumps. Simmer the polenta, stirring often, for 15 minutes. Stir in the grated parmesan and the oil.

Serve the polenta immediately, topped with the meatballs and basil leaves.

nutrition per serve Energy **2060kJ** ‖ Protein **39g** ‖ Fat **19g** (Sat Fat 6g, Poly 2g, Mono 9g)
Carbohydrate **39g** ‖ Fibre **3g**

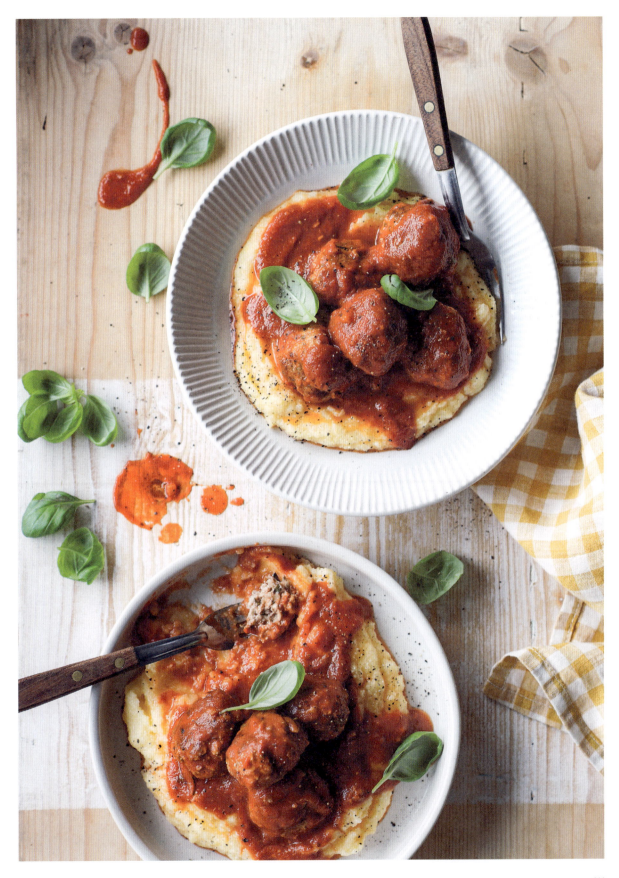

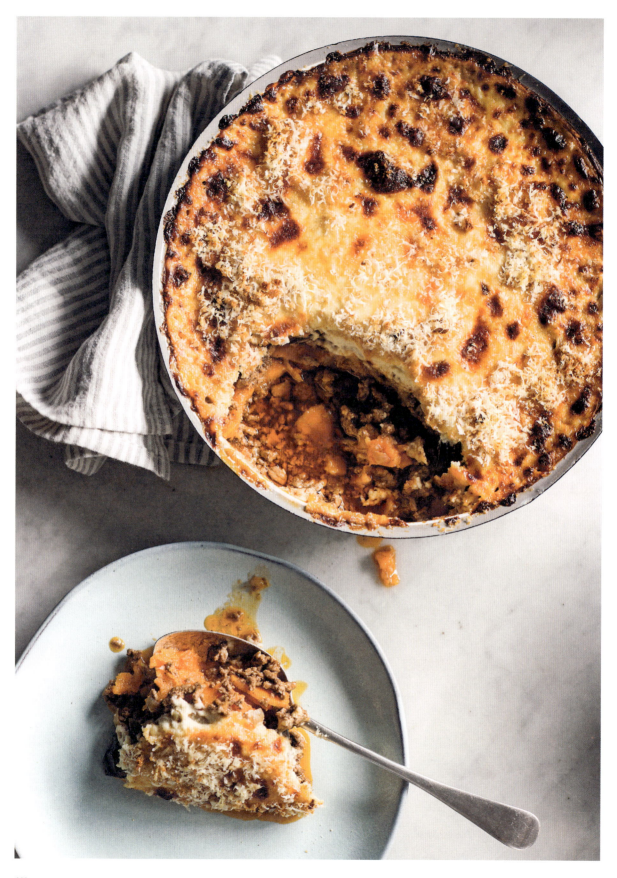

MOUSSAKA

PREP TIME: **40 MINUTES** 🍲 COOK TIME: **1¼ HOURS**

SERVES 6-8

¼ cup (60 ml) extra virgin olive oil
1 large brown onion, finely diced
½ lemon
1 kg lean lamb mince
1 teaspoon ground cinnamon
2 teaspoons dried oregano
½ teaspoon freshly ground
   black pepper
1 tablespoon tomato paste
1 cup (250 ml) dry white wine
2 large eggplant, cut into
   5 mm slices
600 g sweet potato, peeled
   and cut into 5 mm slices

BÉCHAMEL SAUCE

1 tablespoon extra virgin olive oil
¼ cup (35 g) plain flour
3 cups (750 ml) milk
125 g kefalograviera or parmesan
   cheese, grated
½ teaspoon freshly grated nutmeg
1 egg, whisked
½ teaspoon freshly ground
   black pepper
⅓ cup (20 g) fresh wholemeal
   sourdough breadcrumbs

Heat 1 tablespoon of the oil in a large frying pan over medium heat. Sauté the onion until soft, then squeeze the lemon juice over the onion. Add the lamb and fry until brown, stirring to break up the meat. Sprinkle the cinnamon, oregano and black pepper over the lamb and stir through the meat. Stir in the tomato paste, then pour in the wine and cook until the liquid has evaporated, about 5–6 minutes. Remove from the heat and set aside.

Heat a barbecue hotplate or a frying pan to medium heat. Spread 1 tablespoon of the oil over the hotplate or pan. Cook the eggplant slices in batches, turning once, until brown on both sides. Use the remaining tablespoon of oil if needed. Set the eggplant aside on a large tray.

Put the sweet potato in a microwave-safe bowl with a splash of water and cook on High for 5 minutes. Drain and set aside.

To make the béchamel sauce, heat the oil in a saucepan over medium heat. Whisk in the flour and cook for 1 minute. Add a splash of milk and whisk to form a paste. Add a little more milk and continue to whisk into a smooth paste. Gradually add the remaining milk, whisking to combine, then cook until the sauce has thickened. Add all but 25 g of the grated cheese and stir until melted. Sprinkle in half the nutmeg, then slowly add the egg, whisking to combine. Season with the pepper.

Preheat the oven to 180°C. Layer half the eggplant in a deep 30 cm round ovenproof dish. Top with half the lamb mixture, then all of the sweet potato slices. Add the remaining lamb and eggplant. Pour the béchamel sauce over the eggplant and sprinkle with the remaining cheese and breadcrumbs. Bake the moussaka for 45 minutes.

nutrition per serve (8 serves) Energy **2120kJ** ‖ Protein **40g** ‖ Fat **25g** (Sat Fat 8g, Poly 2g, Mono 12g)
Carbohydrate **26g** ‖ Fibre **8g**

MAKE YOUR FRIDGE WORK FOR YOU

How does your fridge look when you open the door? Does it inspire you to eat well, with lots of nutritious options? Is it often bare, with nothing much to eat except a few limp vegies in the crisper drawer? Or is it so jammed full that you can't see what's actually in there?

It's worth making the effort to keep your fridge well organised because a well-ordered fridge helps you to achieve three key aims:

1 Everyone in the family eats better because healthy snacks are in sight and it's so much easier to throw together a quick, nutritious meal when you have the right ingredients to hand.

2 There is less food waste because you can see what is in the fridge and what needs to be used up before it goes off.

3 You save money because less food goes into the bin, you buy what you actually need, and you are more inspired to cook and therefore less likely to resort to takeaway meals.

TIPS FOR ORGANISING YOUR FRIDGE:

→ Store your fruit and vegies in the crisper drawers as this helps to extend their shelf life. Keep your fruit and vegies separate. Fruit gives off ethylene, a natural chemical in the plant involved in ripening the fruit, and this can cause the other produce to spoil faster. Fruit will last longer when stored in a crisper drawer with the humidity control open as far as it will go. This allows ethylene to escape and prevents the fruit from rotting prematurely.
→ Leave unripe tomatoes, avocados, pears, mangoes and other stone fruit on the bench. Once they ripen, transfer them to the fridge, where the cold temperature will dramatically slow the ripening process. Berries, grapes, citrus fruit and apples are all ready to eat when you purchase them and are best kept in the fridge.

- → Wash berries and store them in a container lined with paper towel. Place them on a shelf at kids' eye level next to a tub of natural yoghurt to make this an attractive snack option.
- → Trim and wash leafy greens before spinning them dry in a salad spinner and storing in a reusable storage bag in the crisper drawer. This makes throwing together a quick salad a cinch and you're more likely to get your daily dose of greens. Slide the humidity control all the way closed to help preserve the moisture in the greens and prevent them from wilting.
- → When you're preparing a meal, wash and chop a few extra vegies and store them in reusable containers, ready to use. This will save you preparation time at the next meal. Cut carrots, celery, capsicums and cucumbers into batons, ready to use in lunchboxes or for afternoon tea, along with a healthy dip.
- → Fresh herbs are best washed right before you use them. To preserve bunches of herbs such as parsley, coriander and basil for longer, stand them in a jar of water, place a bag over the leaves and stand upright on a shelf in the fridge. Alternatively, wrap the herbs in beeswax wraps or damp paper towel and store them in a bag in the crisper. Use up herbs that are past their best by blending them into a pesto or salad dressing.
- → Store raw meat, chicken and fish in sealed containers on the bottom shelf of the fridge. This ensures that if there are any leaked juices, they won't contaminate other items in the fridge. Store those that have the shortest shelf life at the front to remind you to use them before they reach their expiry date.
- → Plastic makes cheese 'sweat' and the plastic can leach unwanted chemicals into the cheese. Remove cheese from plastic wrap, rewrap it in baking paper and store it in a container with other cheeses. Soft cheeses such as ricotta, feta, cream cheese and cottage cheese are best left in their original containers, but note that these fresh cheeses have a relatively short shelf life and need to be used quickly.
- → The door of the fridge experiences the greatest fluctuations in temperature, particularly if the fridge is frequently opened. Therefore, the fridge door is a good place to store the most stable items, including mustard, chutney and other condiments, jam, butter, drinks and any nutrition supplements or medications requiring refrigeration. Ensure the latter are out of reach of younger children.
- → It's convenient to store an opened bottle or carton of milk in the fridge door, but store any unopened milk on one of the middle shelves where it is colder, with less temperature fluctuation.
- → Store leftovers in sealed reusable containers ready for easy reheating for the next meal. These should be stored in the middle shelves of the fridge where the temperature is stable.

One of the easiest ways to minimise food waste is to keep your fridge well organised, which means storing your food correctly.

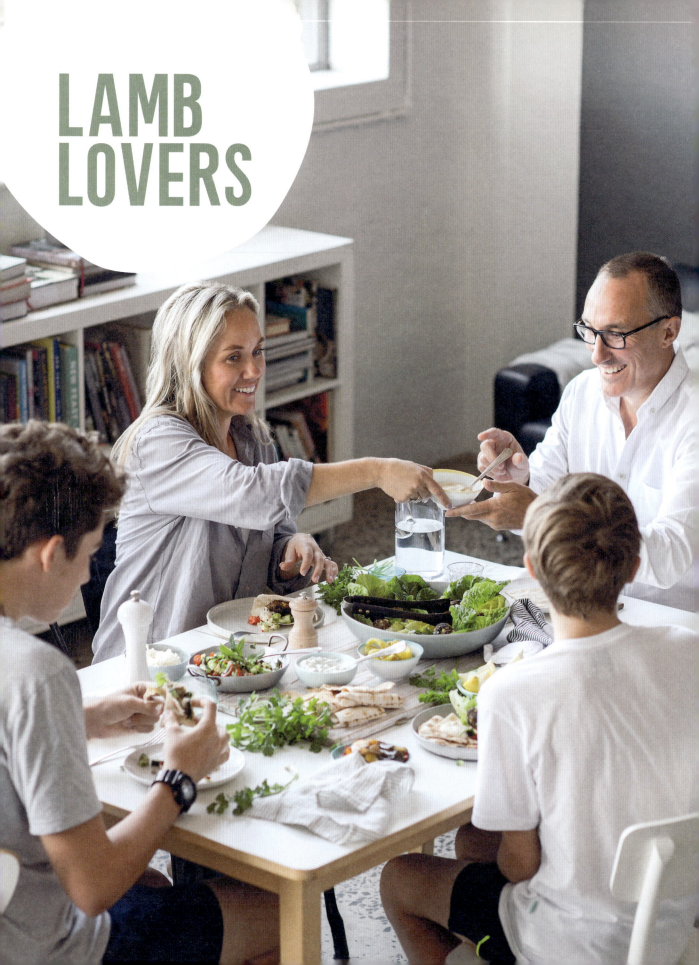

LAMB LOVERS

LAMB KOFTA MEZZE PLATE

PREP TIME: 10 MINUTES 🍵 **COOK TIME: 10 MINUTES**

Don't worry if you're missing an ingredient or two – this style of cooking lends itself to many variations. Serve the koftas with hummus, sauerkraut, marinated roasted vegetables or pickled vegetables, Tomato Salsa Salad (page 89), mixed lettuce leaves and warm wholemeal pita bread.

SERVES 4–6

100 g tinned chickpeas
500 g lamb mince
1 small red onion, finely diced
2 teaspoons ground cumin
½ teaspoon ground cinnamon
½ teaspoon ground turmeric
1 teaspoon garam masala
¼ teaspoon chilli flakes
⅓ cup (70 g) currants
¼ cup (40 g) pine nuts, chopped
½ cup flat-leaf parsley leaves,
    roughly chopped
¼ cup coriander leaves,
    roughly chopped
2 tablespoons mint leaves,
    roughly chopped
Grated zest of 1 lemon
1 tablespoon extra virgin olive oil

MINT YOGHURT
1 cup (260 g) Greek-style yoghurt
1 tablespoon mint leaves, chopped
1 Lebanese cucumber, seeds
    removed, grated
¼ teaspoon ground cumin
¼ teaspoon fine salt

To make the mint yoghurt, mix all the ingredients in a bowl. Refrigerate for 15 minutes to allow the flavours to develop.

Meanwhile, roughly mash the chickpeas with a fork, then transfer to a large bowl. Add the lamb, red onion, spices, currants, pine nuts, herbs and lemon zest. Using your hands, mix the ingredients together.

Shape the lamb mixture into finger-length sausages, about 4 cm thick. Set aside on a tray and refrigerate until required.

Heat a barbecue hotplate, chargrill pan or frying pan to medium. Drizzle the oil over the koftas and cook, turning, for 10 minutes or until cooked through.

Serve the koftas with the mint yoghurt and accompaniments of your choice.

TIPS

→ For a sweeter and more subtle onion flavour, you can sauté the onion in a little extra virgin olive oil until soft and translucent. Allow it to cool before adding it to the mince mixture.
→ You can freeze the raw or cooked koftas.
→ Left-over koftas are great in lunchboxes for school or work.
→ If you're in a hurry, you can use a store-bought tzatziki instead of making the mint yoghurt.

nutrition per kofta Energy **540kJ** ‖ Protein **10g** ‖ Fat **7g** (Sat Fat 1g, Poly 2g, Mono 3g)
Carbohydrate **6g** ‖ Fibre **1g**
(without accompaniments)

SLOW-COOKED LAMB SHOULDER

PREP TIME: **10 MINUTES** COOK TIME: **6 HOURS**

We love this served with roasted pumpkin on a platter of mixed salad leaves, topped with pomegranate tendrils, goat's cheese, almonds, pepitas (pumpkin seeds), parsley and mint, and drizzled with balsamic dressing. Use the left-over lamb to make our fabulous Left-over Lamb and Bean Burritos (see tip, below).

SERVES 8

2.6 kg lamb shoulder, trimmed
  of any thick fat
2 tablespoons extra virgin olive oil
1 teaspoon salt
1 teaspoon freshly ground
  black pepper
1 garlic bulb, skin on, halved
  horizontally
2 brown onions, skin on,
  cut into quarters
1 large carrot, roughly chopped
1 lemon, cut in half
6 thyme sprigs
2 cups (500 ml) chicken stock
1 cup (250 ml) white wine

Preheat the oven to 130°C.

Rub the lamb with the oil and season with the salt and pepper, rubbing it well into the skin. Brown the lamb shoulder in a large deep flameproof casserole dish or an ovenproof frying pan.

Toss the garlic, onions, carrot, lemon halves and thyme sprigs into the frying pan. Pour in the chicken stock and white wine. The liquid should come one-third of the way up the side of the lamb, so add some water, if needed. Cover and bake for 6 hours or until the meat is falling off the bone. Halfway through the cooking time, check that there is enough liquid and add a splash of water if it's drying out.

Shred the lamb, discarding the bone. Drizzle with a little of the cooking juices to help keep the meat moist. Serve with your favourite vegetables.

TIP

→ Chill any left-over lamb in the fridge overnight. Remove any solidified fat from the surface and retain the jus. Discard the garlic and onion skins and thyme stalks. Mix the shredded lamb with the jus, transfer it to an airtight container and freeze to use in Left-over Lamb and Bean Burritos (page 121).

nutrition per serve Energy **1160kJ** ‖ Protein **31g** ‖ Fat **13g** (Sat Fat 4g, Poly 1g, Mono 6g)
Carbohydrate **4g** ‖ Fibre **3g**
(with 100g cooked meat)

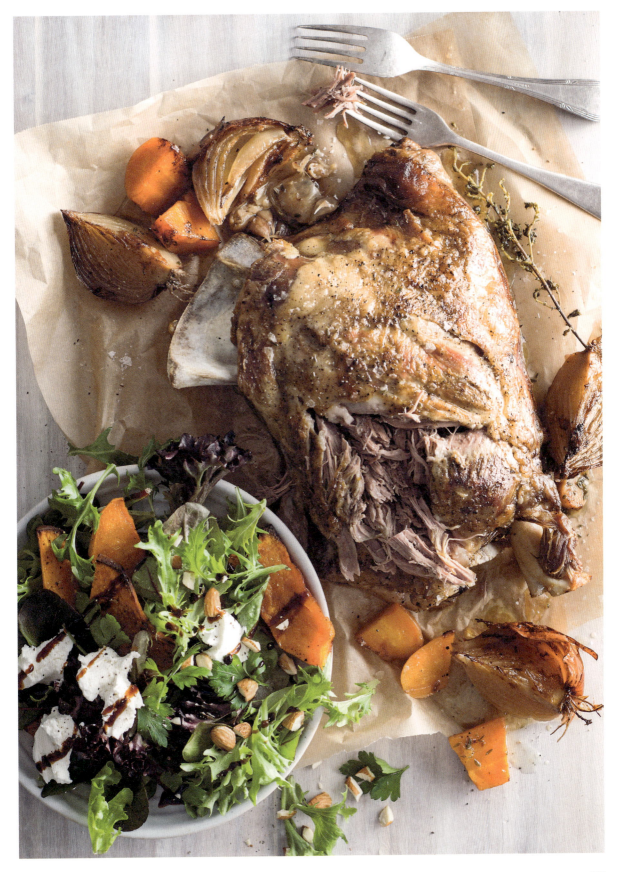

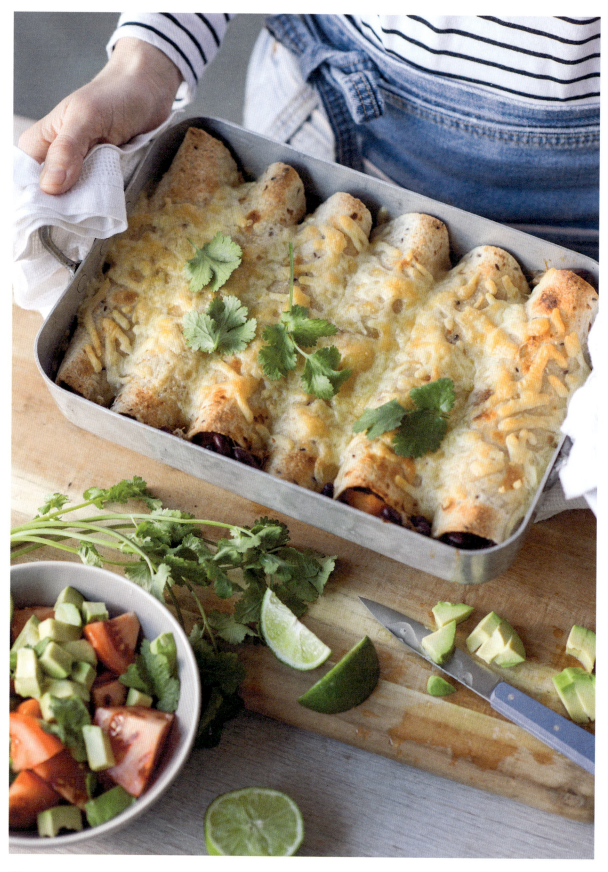

LEFT-OVER LAMB AND BEAN BURRITOS

PREP TIME: 15 MINUTES · **COOK TIME: 20 MINUTES**

This recipe uses the left-over lamb, jus and vegetables from the Slow-cooked Lamb Shoulder on page 118. Serve the burritos with a green salad, a dollop of Greek-style yoghurt, some diced avocado and tomato with a squeeze of lime juice, or our Tomato Salsa Salad (page 89). Active teenagers or bigger men might eat two burritos, hence the recipe makes four to six serves.

SERVES 4-6

500 g cooked left-over lamb, shredded (see page 118)
1 tablespoon ground cumin
2 teaspoons ground coriander
2 teaspoons smoked paprika
½ teaspoon chilli flakes
400 g tin black beans or red kidney beans, drained and rinsed
Extra virgin olive oil, for greasing
6 wholegrain tortillas
100 g cheddar cheese, grated

Heat the lamb and jus in a saucepan over medium heat. You can include the cooked garlic, onion and carrots if you like. Stir in the spices and beans and cook for 2–3 minutes or until the spices are fragrant and the beans are heated through. Turn off the heat and allow the lamb mixture to cool a little.

Preheat the oven to 180°C. Lightly grease a large ovenproof dish with extra virgin olive oil.

Spoon the lamb mixture onto the middle of each tortilla, in a long sausage shape. Fold the sides over the lamb to form a burrito shape.

Place the burritos in the lined dish and sprinkle the cheese over the top. Bake for 10 minutes or until the cheese has melted and the burritos are golden.

nutrition per burrito Energy **2120kJ** ‖ Protein **38g** ‖ Fat **20g** (Sat Fat 8g, Poly 4g, Mono 6g) Carbohydrate **41g** ‖ Fibre **6g**

MINIMISING FOOD WASTE

According to government figures, in Australia one in every five shopping bags of food ends up in the bin. That's estimated to be around $3,800 worth of food per household, per year. If you look at it in terms of a typical household bin, food waste amounts for more than a third of the contents. That's food that ends up rotting in landfill sites, contributing in a major way to greenhouse gas production.

It's pretty shocking when you think about it. Wasting so much food is bad for your wallet and ultimately bad for the planet, not to mention the waste of resources used in producing the food and the packaging that goes along with it. The bottom line is that we all must do more to cut down waste. Below are some tips on how you can minimise food waste at home.

Plan your meals

The more you plan, the less you waste. Conversely, the less you plan, the more likely you are to buy too much food, which will end up in the bin (or to buy takeaway meals!). Even if you don't write out a detailed plan for the week, it's good to have an idea of the key evening meals.

Understand 'best before' and 'use by' dates

A 'use by' date is given when a food must be eaten before a certain time for health or safety reasons. A 'best before' date is a recommendation only – the food is still edible, but it may have lost some quality. Food producers, understandably, want to minimise their risk in foods causing any harm to consumers, so 'best before' dates tend to be very, very safe. However, they undoubtedly lead to more food waste. Compounding the problem is the fact that many consumers think a 'best before' date is the same as a 'use by' date and throw out food even if it's just a day or two past the date. Even a 'use by' date has a safety margin built in, so use your common sense to help you decide whether or not a food is still good to eat.

Store food correctly

It might sound obvious, but storing food correctly will preserve the quality and prolong its shelf life. Check the manufacturer's guide to ensure you are using the crisper drawer of your fridge properly. Always store dry ingredients in sealed, airtight containers. Never store potatoes or onions in the fridge – remove them from plastic bags so that they can breathe, place them in separate baskets or paper bags, then store them in a cool, dark place such as your pantry. Wrap bunches of fresh herbs in damp paper towel and then store them in a reusable sealed bag in the crisper drawer of your fridge. You'll be amazed how much longer they last.

Do a regular fridge and pantry audit

Rather than letting foods go to waste hiding at the back of your fridge or pantry, do a regular clear out and ensure you know exactly what you have. Put foods close to their 'use by' date at the front to encourage them to be eaten. If you can see that you won't get around to eating a particular food in time, consider how else it could be stored – could it be frozen, vacuum sealed or dehydrated?

Consider a food dehydrator

A food dehydrator is a great way to preserve fresh herbs. The dried herbs can be stored in a sealed jar in your pantry for much longer than they will last in the fridge. You can also dry fruit, which is a big hit in kids' lunchboxes or when they are asking for a sweet treat. Some vegies can be dehydrated (some are best blanched prior to drying). And you can even dehydrate lean, cooked meats to make jerky, or dried meat or fish snacks for your dog!

Buy a food vacuum sealer

Vacuum sealers are brilliant for keeping food fresh for longer. By sealing the food and expelling all the air, vacuum sealing can extend the shelf life of fresh foods by about five times. This also means you can buy foods such as meat in bulk, saving you money as well as time. Vacuum sealing food before freezing is also a good idea as it prevents leaking and freezer burn, and the food takes up less space in your freezer.

Cutting down on your family's food waste could be as simple as taking a few minutes to plan your meals for the week.

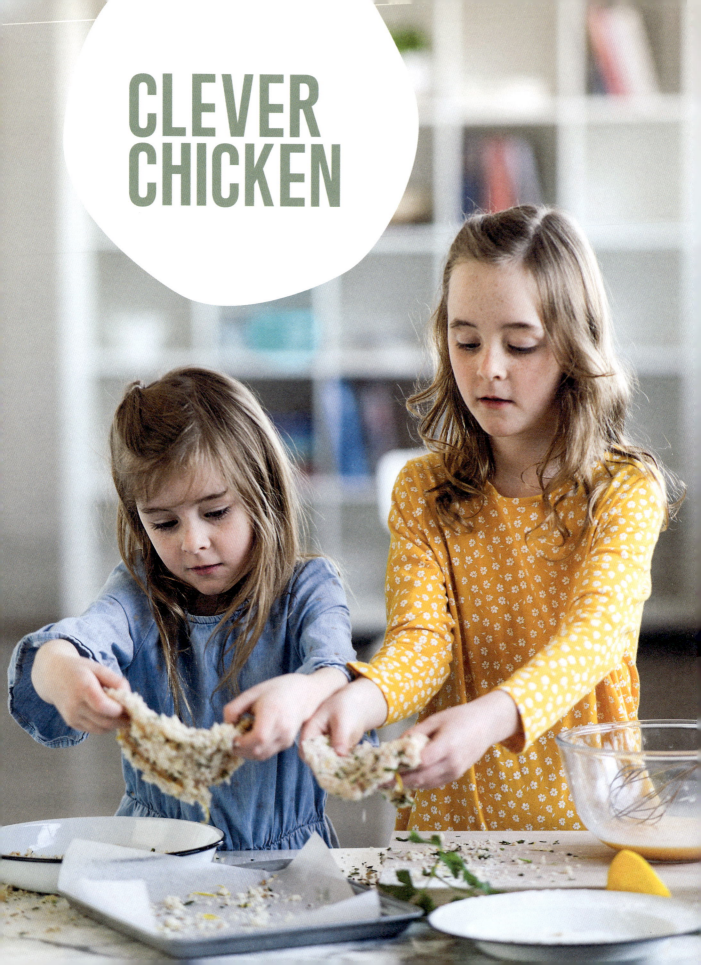

CLEVER CHICKEN

CHICKEN SCHNITZEL

PREP TIME: **10 MINUTES** COOK TIME: **20 MINUTES**

There is no excuse for dull schnitzel – it takes only a few little extras to turn a plain schnitzel crust into a super-tasty schnitzel. Serve it with our Asian Coleslaw (page 98) and Sweet Potato Fries (page 145). Or, for a homemade chicken 'parmie', add a little tomato passata and grated cheese to your pan-fried schnitzel and bake it for 5 minutes.

SERVES 4

- 2 skinless chicken breast fillets or 500 g schnitzel-cut chicken (uncoated)
- 2 cups (120 g) fresh wholegrain sourdough breadcrumbs
- 35 g grated parmesan cheese
- 1 tablespoon flat-leaf parsley leaves, finely chopped, or 1 teaspoon dried parsley
- 1 tablespoon sesame seeds
- ½ teaspoon freshly ground black pepper
- ½ teaspoon grated lemon zest
- 40 g plain flour or cornflour
- 2 large eggs
- 2 tablespoons extra virgin olive oil

Slice each chicken breast in half horizontally. Beat with a meat mallet or a rolling pin until about 5 mm thick.

Combine the breadcrumbs, grated parmesan, parsley, sesame seeds, pepper and lemon zest in a shallow bowl. Put the flour in another shallow bowl. Whisk the eggs in a third shallow bowl.

Dust the chicken in the flour, then dip into the egg, turning to coat. Finally, toss the chicken in the breadcrumb mixture, covering all sides.

Heat the oil in a large frying pan over medium heat. Cook the chicken in batches for 5 minutes on each side or until golden and cooked through. Don't let the pan get too hot otherwise the crumbs will burn. Keep the chicken warm while you cook the remainder.

TIPS

- → You can crumb the chicken ahead and place it on a plate in a single layer, covered with plastic wrap.
- → Use up any stale or left-over bread by making breadcrumbs – blitz the bread in a food processor and store it in an airtight container in the freezer. There's no need to thaw the crumbs before you use them.

nutrition per serve Energy **1670kJ** ‖ Protein **37g** ‖ Fat **19g** (Sat Fat 5g, Poly 3g, Mono 10g) Carbohydrate **18g** ‖ Fibre **2g**

CHICKEN LAKSA WITH SOBA NOODLES

PREP TIME: 10 MINUTES ⟶ **COOK TIME: 20 MINUTES**

It's important to find a laksa paste that you love and trust for this dish. We've tried several and they are definitely not all the same. Asian grocers will offer the best brands – ask for help in choosing which ones taste best.

SERVES 4

- 200 g skinless chicken breast fillet
- 4 large eggs
- 200 g soba noodles
- 200 g jar laksa paste
- 200 ml coconut milk
- 120 g broccolini, stems finely chopped, florets kept whole
- 2 cups (150 g) finely shredded red cabbage
- 150 g baby bok choy, roughly chopped
- 1 cup (115 g) bean sprouts
- 4 baby cucumbers, halved lengthways (optional)
- 2 spring onions, green part only, thinly sliced
- ¼ cup coriander leaves
- 2 tablespoons mint leaves
- 1 lime, cut into wedges

Place the chicken breast and eggs in a small saucepan of water over medium heat. Once the water is boiling, reduce the heat to a simmer and cook the eggs for 8 minutes, then remove with a slotted spoon and run under cold water to cool. Continue to simmer the chicken for a further 2–4 minutes or until cooked through. Turn off the heat and leave the chicken to cool in the liquid for 5 minutes.

Peel the eggs and set aside. Remove the chicken from the liquid and shred the meat with your hands.

Cook the soba noodles according to the packet instructions. Drain and rinse well under cold water.

Whisk the laksa paste, coconut milk and 400 ml water in a saucepan. Bring to a gentle simmer, then add the broccolini and purple cabbage and cook for 1–2 minutes or until the broccolini is just tender. Add the bok choy and cook for 1 minute.

Divide the noodles among four deep bowls. Put the chicken on top of the noodles, then pour in the hot laksa, dividing the vegetables among the bowls. Garnish with the bean sprouts, egg halves, cucumber halves (if using), spring onion, coriander and mint. Serve with the lime wedges.

nutrition per serve   Energy **2130kJ** ‖ Protein **30g** ‖ Fat **19g** (Sat Fat 9g, Poly 3g, Mono 4g)
Carbohydrate **49g** ‖ Fibre **11g**

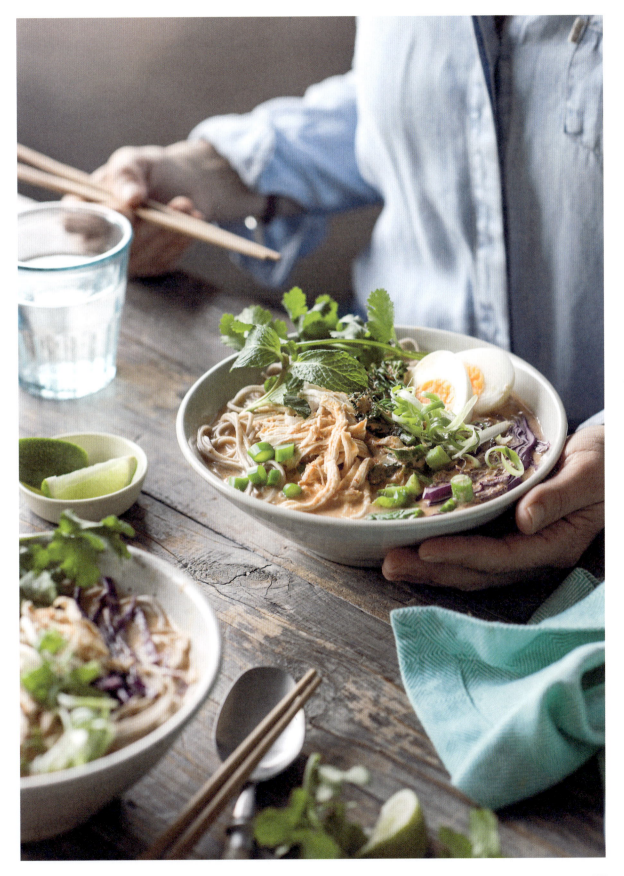

SIMPLE ROAST CHICKEN AND VEG

PREP TIME: **10 MINUTES**   COOK TIME: **1 HOUR 10 MINUTES**

Although roasting a chicken takes a little longer than other cooking methods, it only takes a few minutes of preparation. You can get fancy with stuffings if you like, but our regular roast chicken dinner uses just a lemon in the cavity and a little seasoning. Pop it in the oven, add the vegies a short while later, then go and put your feet up while it cooks.

SERVES 4

2 tablespoons extra virgin olive oil
1 lemon, halved
1 teaspoon smoked paprika
1 teaspoon dried oregano
1.4 kg free-range chicken
2 brown onions, quartered
6 garlic cloves, skin on
2 carrots, scrubbed and cut
    into quarters
4 celery stalks, roughly chopped
240 g pumpkin, skin on,
    cut into 4 wedges
750 g sweet potato, scrubbed
    and cut into large chunks
2 cups (250 g) cauliflower florets
2 thyme sprigs
1 teaspoon salt
1 teaspoon freshly ground
    black pepper
2 teaspoons cornflour

Preheat the oven to 200°C.

Mix 1 tablespoon of the oil with the juice of half the lemon, the paprika and oregano. Rub the mixture over the skin of the chicken. Put both lemon halves into the chicken cavity. Place the chicken, breast side up, on a wire rack in a roasting tin. Roast for about 1 hour or until the juices run clear when you pierce a thigh with a skewer.

Meanwhile, combine all the vegetables in a large roasting tin. Drizzle with the remaining oil and season with the thyme, salt and pepper. Toss to combine. Add the vegetables to the oven about 30 minutes after the chicken.

Once the chicken is cooked, cover it with foil and set aside to rest for 10 minutes. Pour the pan juices into a small saucepan and place over medium–low heat. Mix the cornflour with a little water to form a paste, then add to the pan and stir until the gravy comes to the boil. Taste and check for seasoning.

Slice the chicken and serve with the roast vegies and gravy.

TIP

→ Roast two chickens so that you have plenty of left-over roast meat to use in sandwiches, salads and other dishes.

nutrition per serve   Energy **1930kJ** ‖ Protein **37g** ‖ Fat **14g** (Sat Fat 3g, Poly 2g, Mono 8g)
Carbohydrate **40g** ‖ Fibre **15g**
(with 100g cooked meat)

EGG DROP SOUP WITH COCONUT CORIANDER CHICKEN DUMPLINGS

PREP TIME: **20 MINUTES, PLUS 10 MINUTES SOAKING** COOK TIME: **10 MINUTES**

This is a very rustic soup. You can expect your chicken dumplings to be perfectly imperfect – there's no rolling required. It's a great soup to freeze for a rainy day. Add some noodles for a heartier meal.

SERVES 8

10 g dried shiitake mushrooms
500 g chicken mince
⅓ cup coriander roots, finely chopped
75 g tinned water chestnuts, drained and finely chopped
¼ cup (60 ml) coconut cream
1 spring onion, finely chopped
1 garlic clove, crushed
1 tablespoon grated ginger
Grated zest of 1 lime
8 cups (2 litres) chicken stock
2 tablespoons tamari or light soy sauce
2 tablespoons shaoxing rice wine, dry white wine or sherry
4 large eggs, lightly whisked
3 cups (150 g) baby spinach
Sesame oil, to serve
1 small handful coriander leaves

Soak the mushrooms in a bowl of hot water for 10 minutes, then drain and finely chop.

Add the mushrooms, chicken mince, coriander root, water chestnuts, coconut cream, spring onion, garlic, ginger and lime zest to a large bowl. Mix until thoroughly combined.

Combine the stock, tamari and rice wine in a large saucepan. Bring to the boil, then reduce to a simmer.

Using two teaspoons, scoop out 1 teaspoon of the chicken mixture and use the other spoon to slide the mixture off the spoon and into the simmering stock. Repeat with the remaining chicken mixture. Cook for 2–3 minutes or until the dumplings float to the surface.

Slowly pour in the eggs, stirring continuously for 30 seconds. Add the spinach and stir until wilted.

Serve the soup with a drizzle of sesame oil and a sprinkling of coriander leaves.

nutrition per serve Energy **700kJ** ‖ Protein **17g** ‖ Fat **9g** (Sat Fat 3g, Poly 1g, Mono 3g)
Carbohydrate **4g** ‖ Fibre **1g**

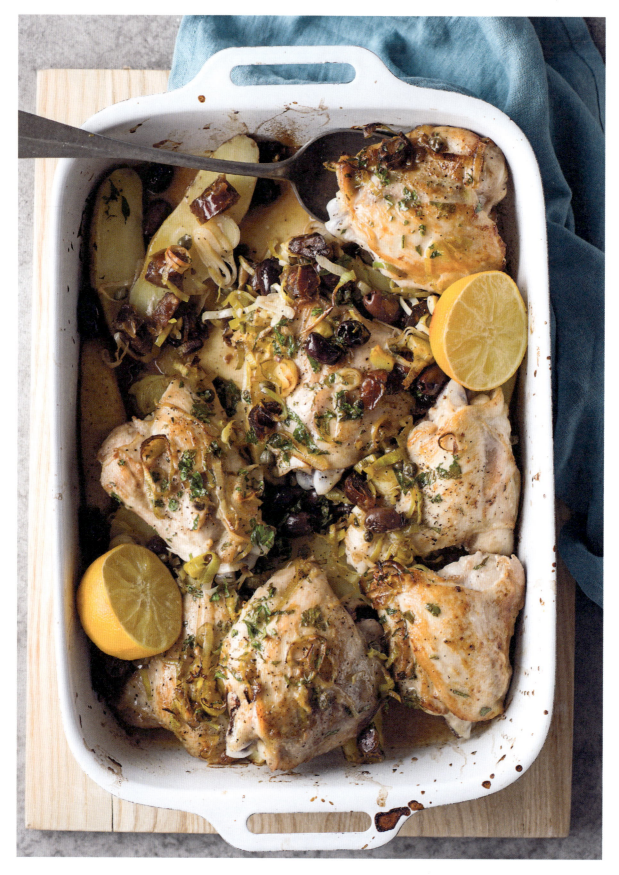

MEDITERRANEAN CHICKEN

PREP TIME: 15 MINUTES 🍲 **COOK TIME: 1 HOUR**

You can make endless variations of this dish, and it works with lots of different vegies. For a one-pot meal, add some asparagus, cherry tomatoes, zucchini, fennel or spinach to the chicken for the last 10 minutes of cooking.

SERVES 4–6

6 kipfler potatoes, skin on, scrubbed

1–2 tablespoons extra virgin olive oil

8 chicken thigh cutlets, bone in and skin removed

1 leek, thinly sliced

1 garlic clove, crushed

4 dates, pitted and roughly chopped

¼ cup (40 g) pitted kalamata olives

½ cup (125 ml) white wine

10 g salted baby capers, rinsed

2 tablespoons flat-leaf parsley leaves, chopped

¼ teaspoon freshly ground black pepper

1 lemon, halved

2 cups (120 g) broccoli florets

4 cups (180 g) shredded silverbeet

Preheat the oven to 180°C.

Cook the potatoes in a large saucepan of boiling water for 10–12 minutes or until just tender. Drain and allow to cool. Cut the potatoes in half lengthways and arrange in a large ovenproof dish.

Heat 1 tablespoon of the oil in a large frying pan over medium heat. Fry the chicken in two batches until brown on both sides. This will take about 10 minutes. Place the browned chicken on top of the potatoes.

Add the leek and garlic to the same frying pan and sauté until softened, about 2–3 minutes. Stir in the dates, olives, wine, capers and parsley, then pour the mixture over the chicken and potatoes. Season with salt and sprinkle with the pepper. Squeeze the lemon juice over the chicken and potatoes and add the lemon halves to the dish. Bake for 30 minutes or until the chicken is cooked through.

Just before serving, microwave, steam or boil the broccoli until tender.

Add the silverbeet to the same frying pan, adding more oil if needed, and sauté for 2–3 minutes or until wilted. Season with a squeeze of lemon from the roasting tin and some salt and freshly ground black pepper.

Serve the broccoli and silverbeet alongside the chicken.

nutrition per serve (4 serves) Energy **1840kJ** ‖ Protein **35g** ‖ Fat **15g** (Sat Fat 3g, Poly 2g, Mono 8g) Carbohydrate **35g** ‖ Fibre **9g**

SOY GINGER CHICKEN

PREP TIME: 5 MINUTES, PLUS 30 MINUTES MARINATING   COOK TIME: **35 MINUTES**

This simple but flavoursome chicken dish is lovely served with brown rice, steamed carrot and zucchini sticks, broccolini and wilted spinach.

SERVES 4

4 x 150 g skinless chicken breast fillets
1 tablespoon extra virgin olive oil
1 tablespoon black or white sesame seeds
Sliced spring onions, to serve

MARINADE

2 cups (500 ml) chicken stock
2 tablespoons tamari or light soy sauce
2 tablespoons shaoxing rice wine or dry white wine
2 garlic cloves, thinly sliced
1 teaspoon grated ginger
½ teaspoon freshly ground black pepper

Mix the marinade ingredients together in a roasting tin. Add the chicken breasts and turn to coat in the marinade. Marinate in the fridge for at least 30 minutes.

Preheat the oven to 180°C.

Heat the oil in a frying pan over medium heat. Transfer the chicken breasts to the pan, leaving the marinade in the roasting tin, and cook for 2–3 minutes on each side or until browned.

Return the browned chicken breasts to the roasting tin and bake for 25–30 minutes or until the chicken is completely cooked through.

Sprinkle the sesame seeds and sliced spring onion over the chicken and serve.

TIP

→ Marinate the chicken the night before (or in the morning) for a quick meal the next night.

nutrition per serve   Energy **950kJ** ∥ Protein **35g** ∥ Fat **7g** (Sat Fat <2g, Poly <2g, Mono 5g)
Carbohydrate **1g** ∥ Fibre **<1g**
(without accompaniments)

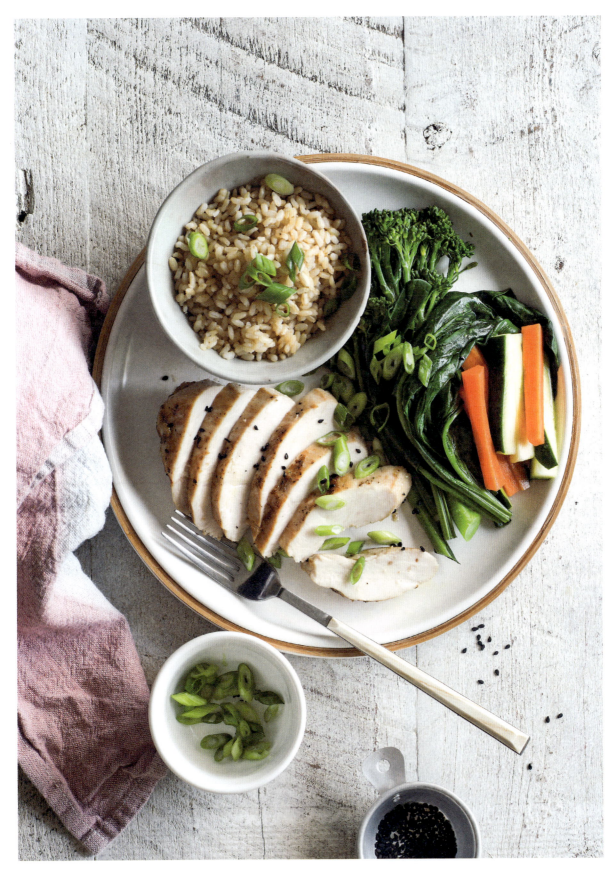

SPICED VEGIE CHICKEN FILO

PREP TIME: **30 MINUTES, PLUS COOLING** COOK TIME: **20 MINUTES**

These tasty chicken and vegie parcels are lovely served with tzatziki or a chunky tomato relish.

MAKES 12

1 small carrot, scrubbed
1 small zucchini
1 celery stalk
60 g pumpkin
½ turnip, peeled
½ brown onion, peeled
¼ cup (60 ml) extra virgin olive oil
½ cup flat-leaf parsley leaves,
   finely chopped
1 teaspoon curry powder
½ teaspoon dried oregano
½ teaspoon salt
½ teaspoon freshly ground
   black pepper
500 g chicken mince
12 sheets filo pastry
1 egg, lightly whisked
1 tablespoon sesame seeds

Grate the carrot, zucchini, celery, pumpkin, turnip and onion in a food processor or using a box grater.

Heat 1 tablespoon of the oil in a frying pan over medium heat. Sauté the grated vegetables and parsley for 2–3 minutes or until soft. Sprinkle with the curry powder and oregano, then season with the salt and pepper. Remove from the heat and transfer to a bowl. Once the vegetables have cooled to room temperature, mix in the chicken.

Preheat the oven to 180°C. Line a large baking tray with baking paper.

Lay a sheet of filo pastry on a clean surface. Brush with some of the remaining oil (it doesn't need to cover the entire sheet). Place a second filo sheet on top, then cut in half lengthways.

Spoon 1 heaped tablespoon of the chicken mixture onto one corner of the pastry strip. Flatten the mixture a little, keeping it to one corner of the pastry. Fold the mixture diagonally to form a triangle, then fold it again in the opposite direction. Continue folding left to right until you reach the end of the strip. Place on the baking tray. Repeat with the second oiled pastry strip.

Repeat the layering, filling and folding process with the rest of the pastry to make 12 triangles in total. Brush the triangles with the egg and sprinkle with the sesame seeds. Bake the parcels for 15 minutes or until the chicken is cooked through and the pastry is golden.

nutrition per serve (2 triangles)   Energy **1360kJ** ‖ Protein **21g** ‖ Fat **17g** (Sat Fat 3g, Poly 2g, Mono 10g)
Carbohydrate **20g** ‖ Fibre **3g**

CHICKEN NAPOLI WITH STEAMED GREENS

PREP TIME: **10 MINUTES** 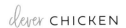 COOK TIME: **35 MINUTES**

*This dish is delicious served over wholegrain spaghetti or brown rice,
or with polenta or Sweet Potato Fries (page 145).*

SERVES 4

1 large garlic clove, peeled
1¼ tablespoons extra virgin olive oil
4 x 125 g skinless chicken breast
  fillets
½ teaspoon salt
400 ml tomato passata
  (puréed tomatoes)
100 g tasty or cheddar cheese,
  grated
2 cups (120 g) broccoli florets
1 large zucchini, cut into batons
2 cups (260 g) frozen peas
2 cups (100 g) baby spinach
Juice of ½ lemon
1 teaspoon za'atar or sesame seeds
½ teaspoon freshly ground
  black pepper

Preheat the oven to 180°C.

Gently bruise the garlic clove with the side of a knife. Heat 1 tablespoon of the oil and the garlic in a frying pan over medium heat. Cook for 2–3 minutes or until the oil is fragrant.

Season the chicken with the salt and a good grinding of black pepper. Cook the chicken in the garlic oil for 3–4 minutes on each side or until golden.

Transfer the chicken to an ovenproof dish. Pour the passata over the chicken and bake for 15–20 minutes. Sprinkle the grated cheese over each chicken breast. Return to the oven for 5 minutes or until the cheese is melted and golden.

Meanwhile, steam the broccoli and zucchini for 5 minutes. Add the peas and baby spinach and steam for 2 minutes or until tender. Alternatively, microwave the vegetables.

Divide the chicken and vegetables among four serving plates. Drizzle the lemon juice and the remaining 1 teaspoon of oil over the vegetables and sprinkle with the za'atar or sesame seeds and freshly ground black pepper.

TIP

→ If you love garlic, you can finely chop the garlic clove once it has infused the oil and include it in the dish. Alternatively, you could use a garlic-infused extra virgin olive oil.

nutrition per serve   Energy **1560kJ** ‖ Protein **41g** ‖ Fat **17g** (Sat Fat 7g, Poly 1g, Mono 7g)
Carbohydrate **10g** ‖ Fibre **8g**

MAKE YOUR FREEZER YOUR FRIEND

Freezing is one of the oldest methods of food preservation. Thousands of years before we had electricity, humans living in colder parts of the world would store food in the snow or in icy caves during the winter months.

Being smart about how you stock and use your freezer can make feeding a busy family so much easier, yet many people don't make the most of their freezer. It becomes little more than a home for ice cream, ice cubes and perhaps some forgotten bread crusts.

From a nutritional perspective, freezing is genius because it means that no preservatives need be added. Another big bonus is that most nutrients are exceptionally well preserved during freezing. Vitamin C is a great example of this – it's readily lost from a plant by exposure to light and air, so that levels in foods such as fresh vegies drop very quickly after picking. In contrast, frozen vegies have been snap frozen on the day they were picked, a process that helps to prevent the plant cell walls from bursting and the vegetables from losing their crunchy texture. This preserves the vitamin C, often resulting in levels that are much higher than in fresh vegies in the supermarket or greengrocers.

TIPS FOR STOCKING AND USING YOUR FREEZER TO MAXIMUM BENEFIT:

→ Keep packets of different frozen vegies so that you can always produce a plant-rich meal, even when you don't have time for a fresh food shop. Individual microwavable packets are really useful when you need to whip up a meal for one.

→ Frozen berries are a terrific source of vitamin C, polyphenols and other beneficial nutrients and phytochemicals. Use them straight from the freezer in fruit smoothies, thaw them to swirl through Greek-style yoghurt for a delicious, easy dessert, or blend them in tangy savoury sauces to serve with a meat or fish dish.

→ Whenever you cook a meal that freezes well, double the recipe and then freeze the extras in individual or family-sized portions for one of those nights you don't have time to cook – or you just don't feel like cooking! Casseroles, curries, bolognese sauce and soups are all ideal for freezing. When making homemade burgers, meatballs or crumbed fish or meat, make extra and freeze them raw.

→ Stock check your fridge and if any meat or fish is getting close to its 'use by' date and you won't get the chance to cook it, pop it into the freezer.

→ Blitz herbs with a little water, pour them into ice cube trays and freeze. You can add these directly to soups, casseroles, stews and sauces. They tend to be much more flavourful than dried herbs.

→ Cook up a big batch of wholegrains such as brown or black rice, quinoa or barley. Divide it into individual or family-sized portions and freeze. This is particularly useful for wholegrains that take a little longer to cook. Simply thaw and reheat in the microwave.

→ When bananas are starting to go brown in the fruit bowl, peel them and pop them into a freezer bag to freeze. Frozen ripe bananas are brilliant for making healthy frozen desserts.

→ Keep an extra loaf or two of sliced wholegrain bread in your freezer. You can toast it directly from the freezer, or thaw slices very quickly on the benchtop, ready for lunchbox sandwiches.

→ When you bake muffins or fruit loaf, individually wrap those you won't use within a couple of days and pop them in the freezer. You can then thaw as required for recess or an afternoon tea snack.

→ Don't ignore the freezer aisle in the supermarket. There are some healthy, nutritious options to have on standby for quick meals, such as ready-marinated or fresh fish fillets, raw or cooked prawns, soups and even some prepared meals. Reading the ingredients list is the easiest way to assess which ones are best. Choose those that list real food ingredients, without added nasties.

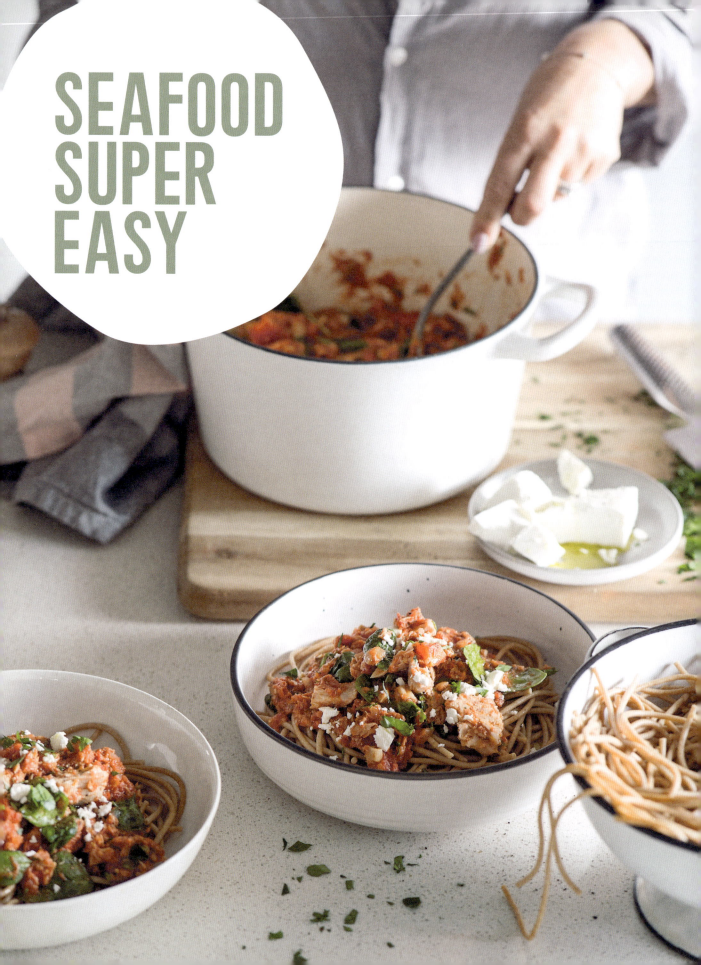

SEAFOOD SUPER EASY

TUNA CHILLI SPAGHETTI

PREP TIME: 10 MINUTES ☕ **COOK TIME: 15 MINUTES**

This pasta dish is probably the one that we both make most regularly. It's so quick to throw together, tastes divine and uses lots of pantry essentials, so it's perfect for when you have very little in the fridge. If you don't have fresh spinach, you can always add a few frozen vegies instead. The sauce is also lovely served on top of a roasted potato or sweet potato with a dollop of Greek-style yoghurt and a sprinkle of parmesan cheese.

SERVES 4

- 400 g wholemeal spaghetti
- 1 tablespoon extra virgin olive oil
- 8 mushrooms (about 200 g), finely diced
- 1 red onion, finely diced
- 1 garlic clove, crushed
- 2 anchovy fillets
- 425 g tin tuna, drained
- 1 bird's eye chilli, finely chopped (optional)
- 2 x 400 g tins no-added-salt crushed tomatoes
- 1 tablespoon flat-leaf parsley leaves, roughly chopped
- 120 g baby spinach
- ½ teaspoon freshly ground black pepper
- 60 g feta cheese or soft goat's cheese, crumbled

Bring a large saucepan of water to the boil. Cook the pasta according to the packet instructions until al dente, then drain.

Meanwhile, heat the oil in a large frying pan over medium heat. Sauté the mushrooms, onion, garlic and anchovies until softened. Stir in the tuna and chilli, if using. Add the tomatoes and parsley. Gently simmer for 10 minutes or until the sauce has thickened slightly.

Stir in the spinach and season with the black pepper.

Stir the pasta through the sauce or divide the pasta among serving bowls and top with the sauce. Serve sprinkled with the crumbled feta.

TIPS

→ If your family really don't like wholemeal pasta, look for high-fibre white pasta, which is available in most supermarkets.
→ If you're using goat's cheese, you can add it with the spinach and cook, stirring, until it has melted into the sauce.

nutrition per serve   Energy **2440kJ** ‖ Protein **38g** ‖ Fat **13g** (Sat Fat 4g, Poly 2g, Mono 5g)
Carbohydrate **68g** ‖ Fibre **16g**

FISH TACOS

PREP TIME: **10 MINUTES, PLUS 20 MINUTES MARINATING** COOK TIME: **6 MINUTES**

Trout is a fabulous source of long-chain omega-3 fats, essential for brain health, brain development and heart health. Family members with higher energy requirements, such as active teenagers and men, will need two tacos, so scale this recipe up or down to suit your family. You can also use salmon fillets.

MAKES 6

600 g ocean or rainbow trout
  fillets, skin on
2 teaspoons red curry paste
2 tablespoons coconut cream
1 teaspoon fish sauce
1 teaspoon pure maple syrup
Juice of ½ lime
Extra virgin olive oil, for drizzling
6 x 40 g wholemeal tortillas,
  warmed
Tomato Salsa Salad (page 89)
2 cups (80 g) lettuce leaves,
  shredded
½ cup (130 g) Greek-style yoghurt
Lime or lemon wedges, to serve

Put the trout in a large bowl. Combine the curry paste, coconut cream, fish sauce, maple syrup and lime juice in a bowl. Pour the curry mixture over the trout and marinate for at least 20 minutes.

Heat a barbecue hotplate or a frying pan to medium heat. Drizzle a little of the oil over the hotplate or pan. Cook the trout, skin side down, for 2–3 minutes on each side or until done to your liking. Remove from the heat and roughly flake the trout into a bowl. Discard the skin.

Put the trout, warm tortillas, salad, shredded lettuce, yoghurt and lime or lemon wedges in the centre of the table and let everyone assemble their own taco.

TIPS

→ Use a mild curry paste for those who don't like their food too spicy. For toddlers and younger children, serve the trout with a little brown rice or quinoa and a dollop of yoghurt, and a few salad vegies on the side.
→ Use any left-over trout in a lunchbox salad. It's also great on a crusty wholegrain sourdough baguette with fresh herbs, tomato, grated carrot, lettuce and a little whole-egg mayonnaise.

nutrition per taco Energy **1620kJ** ‖ Protein **26g** ‖ Fat **19g** (Sat Fat 6g, Poly 3g, Mono 7g)
Carbohydrate **25g** ‖ Fibre **5g**

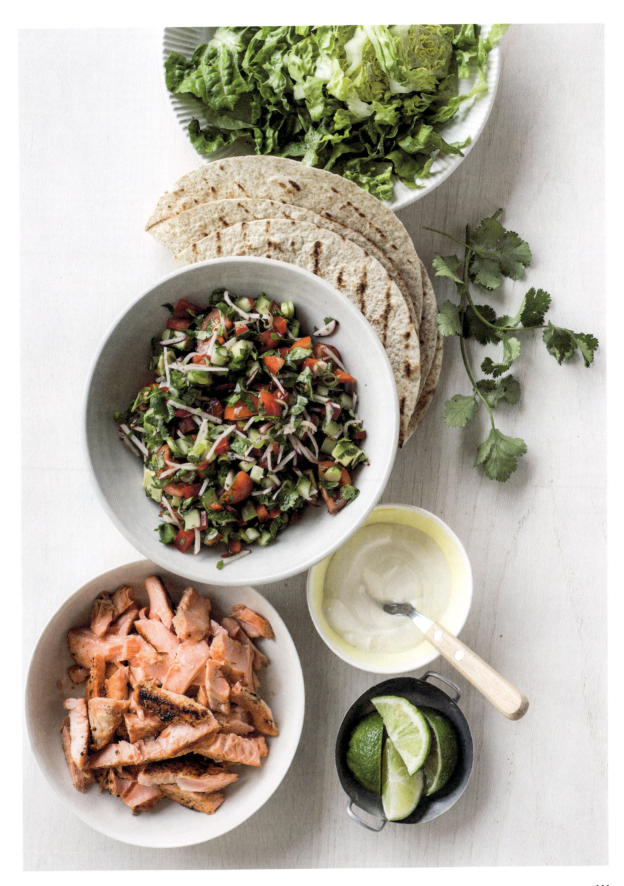

PUMPKIN, CHICKPEA AND FISH CURRY

PREP TIME: **10 MINUTES** COOK TIME: **35 MINUTES**

Serve this tasty curry with brown rice or quinoa and a side of steamed greens, such as broccoli or Asian greens. Or add the vegetables to the curry – use kale, Tuscan cabbage, beans, peas, bean sprouts... whatever vegetables you have in the fridge.

SERVES 6

1 tablespoon extra virgin olive oil
1 brown onion, finely diced
Pinch of salt
1 garlic clove, crushed
3 cm piece ginger, peeled
    and grated
1 tablespoon ground cumin
2 teaspoons ground coriander
1 teaspoon ground turmeric
1 teaspoon ground chilli (optional)
800 g peeled pumpkin,
    cut into 3 cm cubes
400 g tin chickpeas, drained
    and rinsed
2 cups (500 ml) chicken or
    vegetable stock
500 g skinless white fish fillets,
    such as blue eye or ling,
    cut into large cubes
12 raw king prawns, peeled
    and deveined, tails intact
½ cup coriander leaves,
    roughly chopped
120 g baby spinach
Juice of 1 lime

Heat the oil in a frying pan over medium heat. Add the onion and salt and sauté for 2–3 minutes or until the onion starts to soften. Add the garlic and ginger and cook for 1 minute. Add the spices and fry for 1 minute to release their aroma.

Stir in the pumpkin, chickpeas and stock. Cover and cook for 25 minutes.

Add the fish cubes and cook for another 2–3 minutes. Add the prawns and simmer for 2–3 minutes or until the seafood is cooked. Stir in the coriander and spinach.

Taste and season with lime juice, a little salt and freshly ground black pepper.

TIP

→ A grain cooker makes it super easy to cook brown rice, quinoa and other grains perfectly every time. Cook more than you need and freeze the extra for a quick meal another day.

nutrition per serve Energy **1090kJ** Protein **29g** Fat **6g** (Sat Fat <1g, Poly 1g, Mono 3g)
Carbohydrate **18g** Fibre **7g**

TUNA AND SPINACH CURRY WITH BOILED EGGS

PREP TIME: **10 MINUTES** COOK TIME: **15 MINUTES**

This is a go-to recipe for those weeknights when you need to put food on the table fast and with minimal fuss. We use microwavable ready-cooked brown rice for convenience, but you could also use rice that you've cooked yourself and stored in the freezer or, of course, cook it from scratch if you have time.

SERVES 4

3 large eggs
1 tablespoon extra virgin olive oil
1 small onion, finely chopped
425 g tin tuna in springwater
2 cups (500 ml) milk
1 tablespoon plain flour
1 tablespoon curry powder
Grated zest of 1 lemon
3 cups (180 g) broccoli florets
4 cups (200 g) baby spinach
2 x 250 g microwavable pouches
   cooked brown rice
Lemon quarters, to serve

Bring a small saucepan of water to the boil. Gently add the eggs and cook for 7–8 minutes for hard-boiled eggs. Remove from the heat and drain.

While the eggs are cooking, heat the oil in a frying pan over medium heat. Sauté the onion until soft and translucent.

Drain the tuna, reserving the springwater. Mix the milk and springwater together in a jug.

Stir the flour and curry powder into the sautéed onion. Pour in a quarter of the milk mixture, whisking to remove lumps, and cook over medium heat for 2–3 minutes or until the sauce thickens. Stir in the remaining milk mixture, then stir in the lemon zest and tuna and mix well.

Put the broccoli in a microwave-safe bowl with a splash of water and cook on High for 2–3 minutes or until tender but still crunchy.

Peel and slice the eggs. Fold into the curry along with the spinach. Cook for 1–2 minutes until the spinach has wilted.

Heat the rice according to the packet instructions, then divide it among serving bowls and top with the tuna curry. Serve with the broccoli and lemon wedges on the side.

nutrition per serve Energy **1980kJ** ‖ Protein **35g** ‖ Fat **13g** (Sat Fat 4g, Poly 2g, Mono 6g)
Carbohydrate **49g** ‖ Fibre **7g**

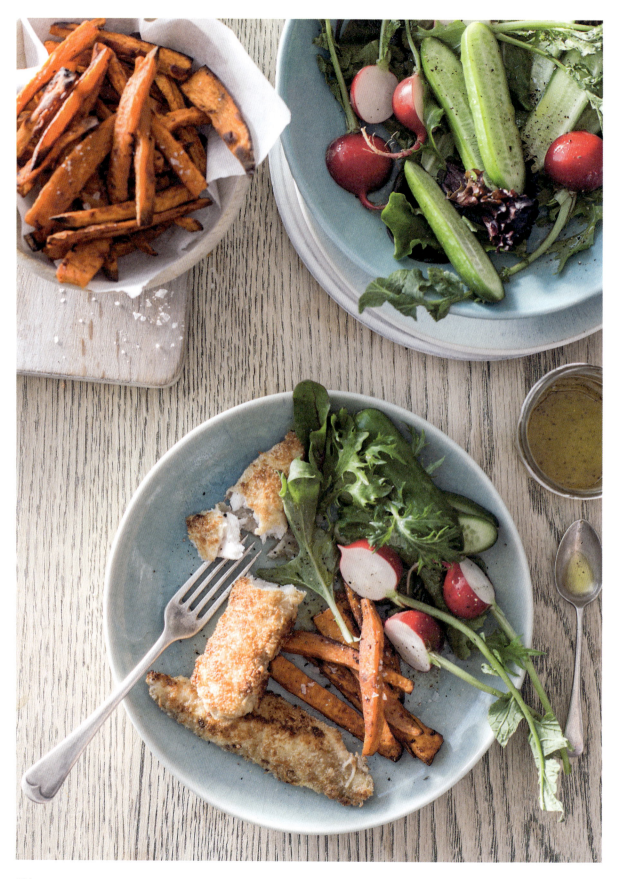

COCONUT FISH FINGERS WITH SWEET POTATO FRIES

PREP TIME: 15 MINUTES **COOK TIME: 40 MINUTES**

Serve the fish with the fries and a lovely big salad of mixed greens and other vegies dressed with one of the salad dressings from pages 104–105.

SERVES 4

800 g sweet potatoes, scrubbed, skin on
2 tablespoons extra virgin olive oil
1 teaspoon smoked paprika
400 g flathead fillets (or any firm white fish)
1 cup (60 g) fresh wholemeal sourdough breadcrumbs
2 tablespoons shredded or desiccated coconut
¼ cup (50 g) semolina
¼ cup (35 g) plain flour
2 large eggs
Salt flakes

Preheat the oven to 200°C. Line a large baking tray with baking paper.

Cut the sweet potatoes into large, long matchsticks and place in a large bowl. Toss with 1 tablespoon of the oil and sprinkle with the paprika and freshly ground black pepper. Spread the fries on the tray in a single layer. Bake for about 40 minutes, flipping halfway through the cooking time, or until the fries are browned and cooked through. Don't worry if the edges of the fries become slightly darkened.

While the fries are cooking, cut the flathead fillets into fingers (one fillet will make approximately three fish fingers).

Combine the breadcrumbs, coconut and semolina in a shallow bowl. Season with freshly ground black pepper. Put the flour in another shallow bowl. Whisk the eggs in a third shallow bowl.

Dust the fish in the flour, then dip into the egg, turning to coat. Finally, toss the fish in the breadcrumbs, covering all sides.

Heat the remaining 1 tablespoon of oil in a large frying pan over medium–low heat. Cook the fish, turning, until golden and cooked through, about 8–10 minutes. Don't let the pan get too hot otherwise the crumbs will burn.

Remove the fries from the oven and sprinkle with a little salt. Serve immediately with the fish fingers.

nutrition per serve Energy **2020kJ** ‖ Protein **32g** ‖ Fat **16g** (Sat Fat 5g, Poly 2g, Mono 8g)
Carbohydrate **49g** ‖ Fibre **8g**

SAFFRON LEMONGRASS MUSSELS

PREP TIME: **10 MINUTES** COOK TIME: **10 MINUTES**

Mussels are such a winning food from both nutritional and environmental perspectives. They're fabulously rich in iron and zinc (great if you have a non-meat eater in the family who will eat shellfish) and they are a sustainable seafood. The added bonus is that they're cost effective and fantastically quick to cook. Don't be scared to give them a shot – you might be surprised how many kids actually like them.

SERVES 2

1 tablespoon extra virgin olive oil

1 large leek, sliced

2 lemongrass stems, pale part only, finely chopped

2 garlic cloves, thinly sliced

2 tablespoons coriander roots, washed and finely chopped

Pinch of saffron threads

½ teaspoon cayenne pepper

1 teaspoon curry powder

1 green chilli, seeded and thinly sliced (optional)

2 kg mussels, scrubbed and de-bearded

1 cup (250 ml) white wine

1 baby cos or butter lettuce, shredded

½ teaspoon freshly ground black pepper

½ Lebanese cucumber, finely diced

10 Thai basil or coriander leaves, shredded

Lime or lemon wedges, to serve

8 slices crusty wholegrain sourdough, toasted

Heat the oil in a large saucepan over medium heat. Add the leek, lemongrass, garlic, coriander root, saffron, cayenne pepper, curry powder and chilli, if using, and sauté until soft, about 5 minutes.

Add the mussels to the pan and place a lid on top. Cook for 2–3 minutes, shaking the pan to stimulate the mussels to open.

Add the white wine and shredded lettuce, shaking the pan again. Season with the pepper and a pinch of salt.

Transfer the mussels to serving bowls and sprinkle with the cucumber and shredded basil or coriander. Serve with lime or lemon wedges and toasted bread to mop up the juices.

TIP

→ Traditional advice was to discard any mussels that don't open on cooking. The thought was that such mussels were dead before cooking and may be unsafe to eat. This has now been disproven. Sydney Fish Market advises prying open any closed mussels. If they smell good, they are good to eat. You should discard any mussels that are open before cooking and don't close with a gentle tap – these mussels are no longer alive and should not be cooked.

nutrition per serve Energy **1580kJ** ‖ Protein **34g** ‖ Fat **10g** (Sat Fat 1g, Poly 2g, Mono 4g)
Carbohydrate **38g** ‖ Fibre **7g**

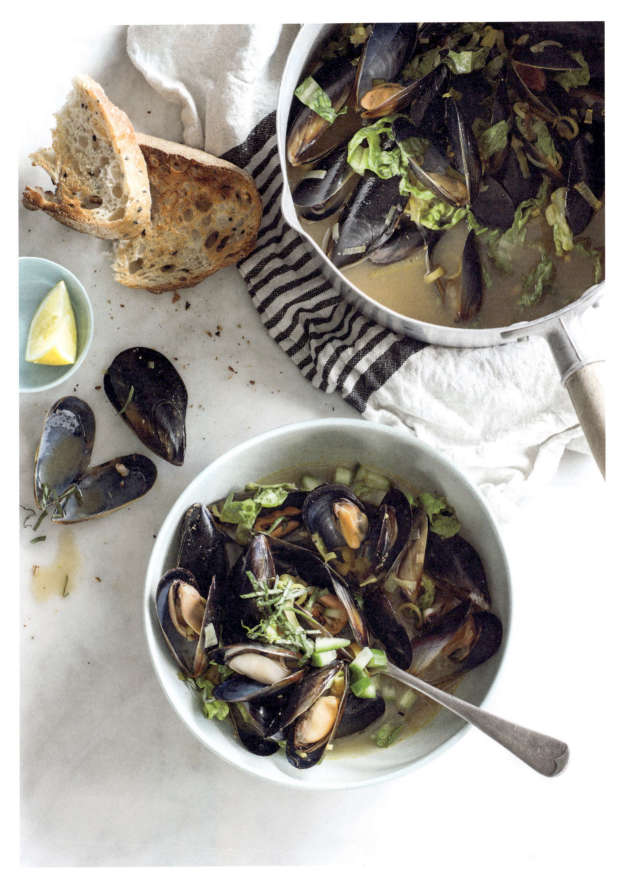

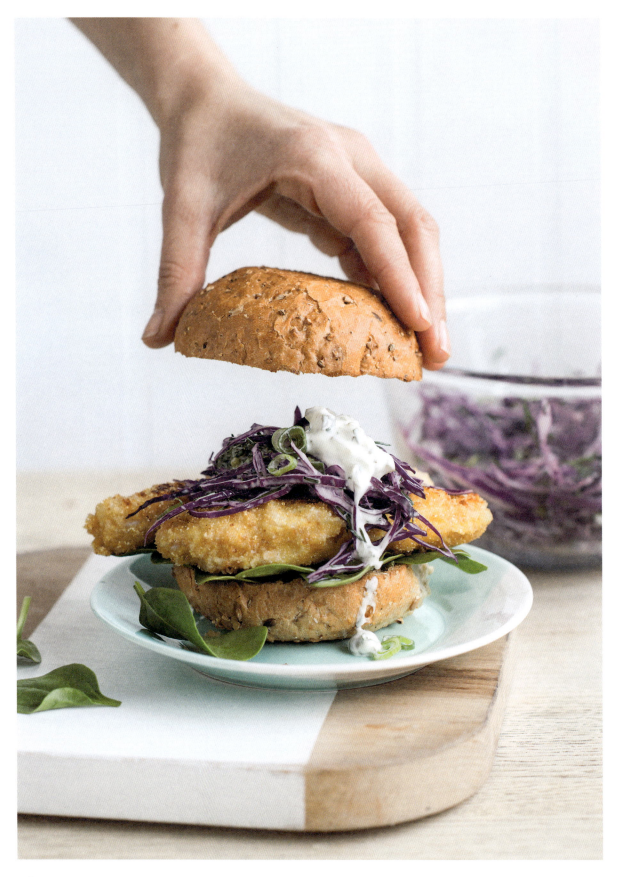

FISH BURGERS WITH COLESLAW

PREP TIME: **20 MINUTES** COOK TIME: **10 MINUTES**

SERVES 4

85 g fresh wholemeal sourdough breadcrumbs
¼ cup (40 g) polenta
¼ cup (20 g) grated parmesan cheese
⅓ cup (50 g) plain flour
2 large eggs
250 g firm white fish fillets, cut into long strips
1 tablespoon extra virgin olive oil
2 cups (100 g) baby spinach
4 wholemeal seed rolls

YOGHURT TARTARE SAUCE

¼ cup (60 g) Greek-style yoghurt
25 g dill pickles, finely chopped
1 teaspoon salted baby capers, rinsed and chopped
1 tablespoon flat-leaf parsley leaves, finely chopped
2 teaspoons lemon juice

COLESLAW

2 cups (150 g) finely shredded red cabbage
1 spring onion, finely chopped
1 tablespoon mint leaves, shredded
1 tablespoon dill, chopped
½ green chilli, thinly sliced
1 tablespoon whole-egg mayonnaise
2 teaspoons white wine vinegar

To make the yoghurt tartare sauce, mix the yoghurt, pickles, capers, parsley and lemon juice in a small bowl. Season with freshly ground black pepper. Refrigerate until needed.

To make the coleslaw, toss the cabbage with the spring onion, herbs and chilli. Whisk the mayonnaise and vinegar, then toss through the cabbage mixture. Season with freshly ground black pepper. Refrigerate until needed.

Combine the breadcrumbs, polenta and parmesan in a shallow bowl. Put the flour in another shallow bowl. Whisk the eggs in a third shallow bowl.

Dust the fish in the flour, then dip into the egg, turning to coat. Finally, toss the fish in the breadcrumb mixture, covering all sides.

Heat the oil in a large frying pan over medium heat. Cook the crumbed fish, turning, until golden and cooked through, about 8–10 minutes. Don't let the pan get too hot otherwise the crumbs will burn.

Serve the fish with the spinach, coleslaw and yoghurt tartare on a lovely wholemeal seeded roll.

TIP

→ We like to toast the rolls on the inside only, leaving the outside soft. Do this by toasting the cut sides of the rolls under the oven grill for 2–3 minutes, just before assembling the burgers.

nutrition per serve   Energy **2260kJ** ‖ Protein **32g** ‖ Fat **17g** (Sat Fat 4g, Poly 4g, Mono 7g)
Carbohydrate **60g** ‖ Fibre **9g**

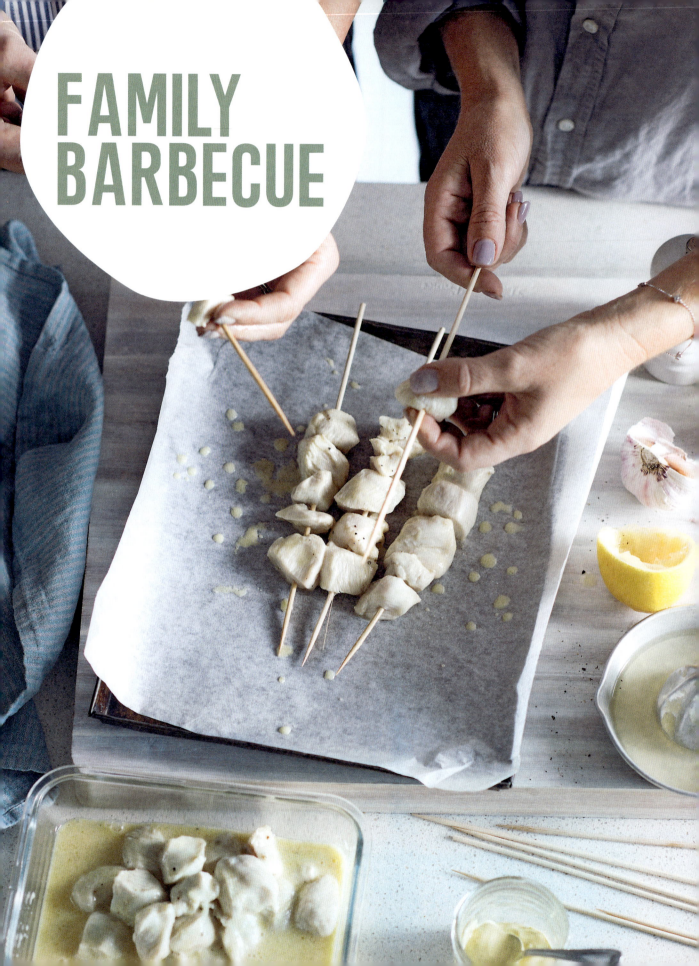

FAMILY
BARBECUE

LEMON MUSTARD CHICKEN SKEWERS

PREP TIME: 10 MINUTES, PLUS 15 MINUTES MARINATING COOK TIME: **10 MINUTES**

This chicken is great served in wholemeal tortilla wraps. Add your choice of coleslaw, Greek-style yoghurt, hummus, avocado, cheese, kimchi or lettuce.

SERVES 4

400 g skinless chicken breast fillets
¼ cup (60 ml) extra virgin olive oil
Juice of 1 lemon
1 tablespoon dijon mustard
1 garlic clove, crushed
½ teaspoon ground black pepper
Pinch of salt flakes

Cut the chicken into 2 cm cubes and place it in a glass dish.

Whisk the remaining ingredients together. Pour the marinade over the chicken and leave to marinate for at least 15 minutes.

Meanwhile, soak eight bamboo skewers in water for 10 minutes.

Heat a barbecue hotplate or chargrill pan to medium. Thread the chicken onto the skewers and cook, turning, for 10 minutes or until the chicken is cooked through.

TIP

→ When you're short on time, don't worry about marinating the chicken for 15 minutes. Just mix the chicken with the marinade and thread onto the skewers, basting with the marinade while it's cooking. Alternatively, you can marinate the chicken the night before or in the morning, ready for dinner that night.

nutrition per serve (2 skewers) Energy **990kJ** ‖ Protein **23g** ‖ Fat **16g** (Sat Fat 3g, Poly 2g, Mono 11g)
Carbohydrate **<1g** ‖ Fibre **<1g**

TAMARI LAMB SKEWERS

PREP TIME: 10 MINUTES, PLUS 15 MINUTES MARINATING   **COOK TIME: 10 MINUTES**

*Buy some ready-shredded vegies and make a yoghurt-based dressing
(see page 163), and add some warm wholemeal tortillas and lime wedges
for a quick and easy meal.*

SERVES 4

400 g lamb backstraps
50 ml red wine vinegar
2 tablespoons extra virgin olive oil
1 tablespoon tamari or light
  soy sauce
1 teaspoon dijon mustard
½ teaspoon ground black pepper

Soak eight bamboo skewers in water for 10 minutes. Cut the lamb backstraps into 3 cm cubes and thread onto the skewers. Place the lamb skewers in a glass dish.

Combine the remaining ingredients. Pour the marinade over the lamb and leave to marinate for at least 15 minutes.

Heat a barbecue hotplate or chargrill pan to medium. Cook the skewers, turning regularly, for about 10 minutes or until they are done to your liking.

TIP

→ Avoid cooking meat on a very high heat as this burns the outside of the meat and can produce potentially carcinogenic compounds. The risk is greatly reduced by using marinades and turning down the heat to gently cook the meat.

nutrition per serve (2 skewers) Energy **520kJ** ‖ Protein **20g** ‖ Fat **4g** (Sat Fat 1g, Poly <0.5g, Mono 2g)
Carbohydrate **<1g** ‖ Fibre **0g**
(without accompaniments)

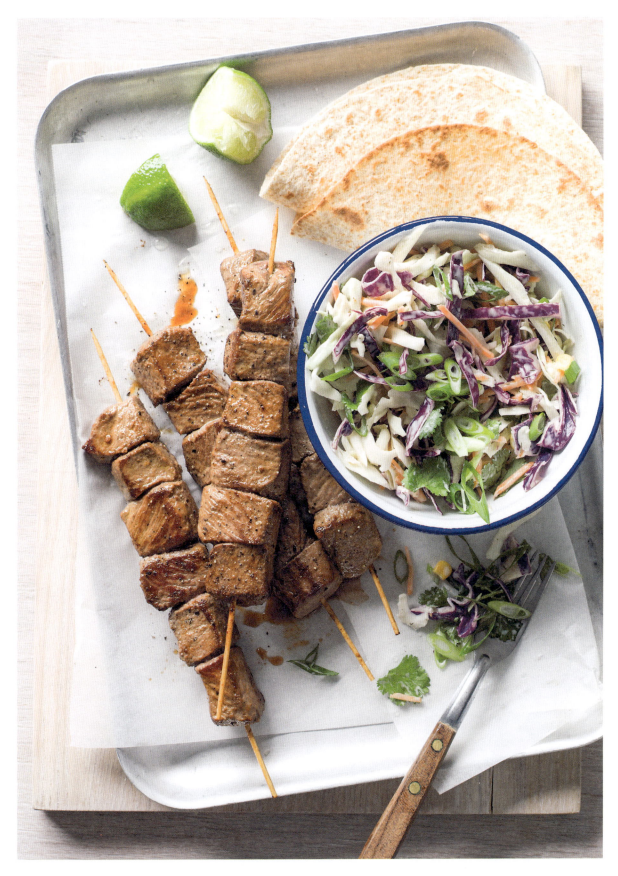

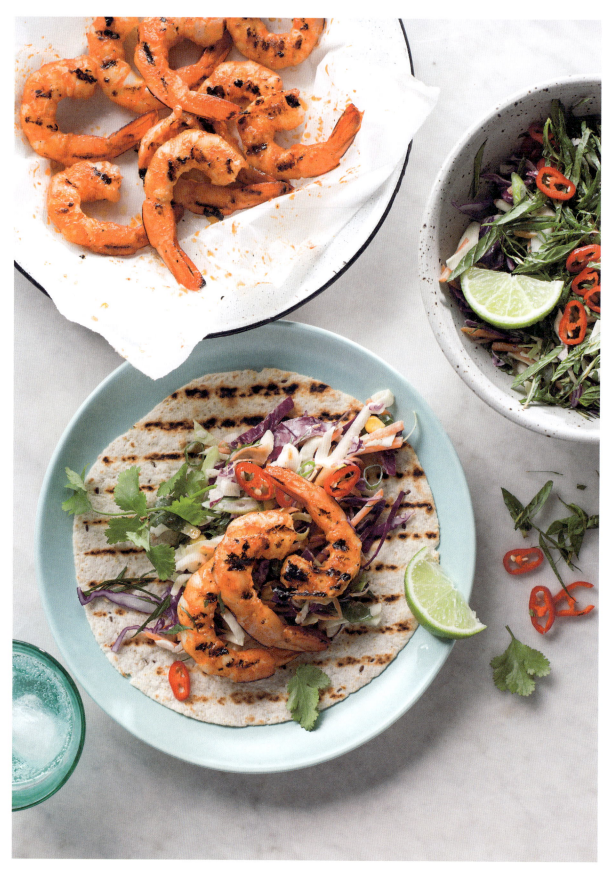

BARBECUED CHILLI PRAWNS

PREP TIME: 5 MINUTES, PLUS 30 MINUTES MARINATING **COOK TIME: 5 MINUTES**

The simplest recipes are almost always the best. And these prawns, as simple as they are, are truly delish! We like to serve them with Mango, Avocado, Bocconcini and Radicchio Salad (page 95) and steamed brown rice. You could also serve them in soft tacos using wholegrain tortillas and a yoghurt-dressed coleslaw.

SERVES 4 AS A STARTER

12 raw king prawns
1 tablespoon hot chilli sauce
1 tablespoon extra virgin olive oil
1 teaspoon pure maple syrup

Peel and devein the prawns, leaving the tails intact. Put the prawns in a large bowl.

Whisk the chilli sauce, oil and maple syrup together in a bowl. Pour the marinade over the prawns and marinate in the fridge for at least 30 minutes.

Heat a barbecue hotplate or grill or a chargrill pan to high. Cook the prawns for 2 minutes on each side or until just cooked through. Serve immediately.

TIP

→ While young children might not like chilli, many older children do. Don't be scared to let them try new tastes. They'll never develop a more adventurous palate if they're only ever given 'kids' food'!

nutrition per serve   Energy **430kJ** ‖ Protein **12g** ‖ Fat **5g** (Sat Fat <1g, Poly <1g, Mono 3g)
Carbohydrate **2g** ‖ Fibre **<1g**
(without accompaniments)

BARBECUED BEEF WITH SESAME GINGER DRESSING

PREP TIME: **5 MINUTES, PLUS 30 MINUTES MARINATING** COOK TIME: **10–15 MINUTES**

Marinating meat before you barbecue it lifts your meal from simple to delicious. We've used Asian-inspired flavours to pair with the beef. We favour cooking one or two large rump steaks and then slicing them, but you can also cook individual steaks. Alternatively, when entertaining and feeding more than four people, check out our tip for cooking a half or whole beef fillet.

SERVES 4

600 g beef fillet steak or
   rump steak
1 teaspoon sesame seeds

MARINADE

1 tablespoon shaoxing rice wine,
   dry white wine or sherry
1 tablespoon rice wine vinegar
1 tablespoon extra virgin olive oil
½ teaspoon sesame oil
1 tablespoon finely chopped
   coriander root
1 teaspoon finely grated ginger
1 garlic clove, finely chopped
1 bird's eye chilli, finely chopped

Put the beef in a large glass bowl. Mix all of the marinade ingredients together. Pour the marinade over the beef and allow it to marinate for at least 30 minutes.

Heat a barbecue hotplate or grill or a chargrill pan to high. Sear the beef for 4–6 minutes on each side or until done to your liking.

Thinly slice the beef, then sprinkle with the sesame seeds and serve with a green salad and steamed brown rice or soba noodles.

TIP

→ To cook a 1–1.5 kg half or whole fillet of beef, sear the beef on all sides, then move it away from the direct heat and close the lid of the barbecue. The cooking time will vary depending on the thickness of the beef, but a rough guide is 15–25 minutes. Beef fillet is very lean, so take care not to overcook it or it will be tough and dry. It's best served rare or at least a little pink in the middle. Transfer the beef to a warm plate and cover it with foil to rest for 5–10 minutes before slicing. It will continue to cook while it's resting, so remove it from the heat just before it's ready.

nutrition per serve   Energy **1090kJ** ‖ Protein **34g** ‖ Fat **13g** (Sat Fat 4g, Poly 2g, Mono 7g)
Carbohydrate **<1g** ‖ Fibre **<1g**
(without accompaniments)

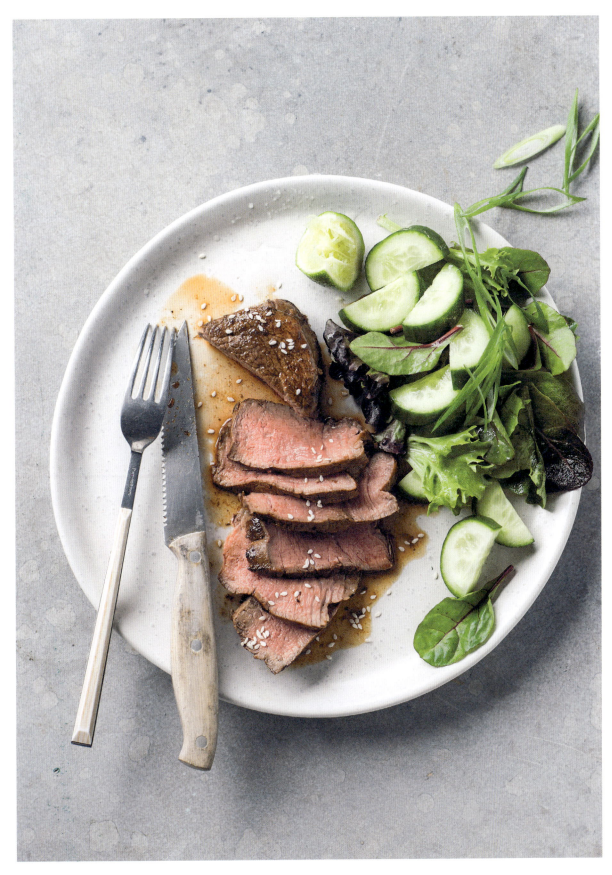

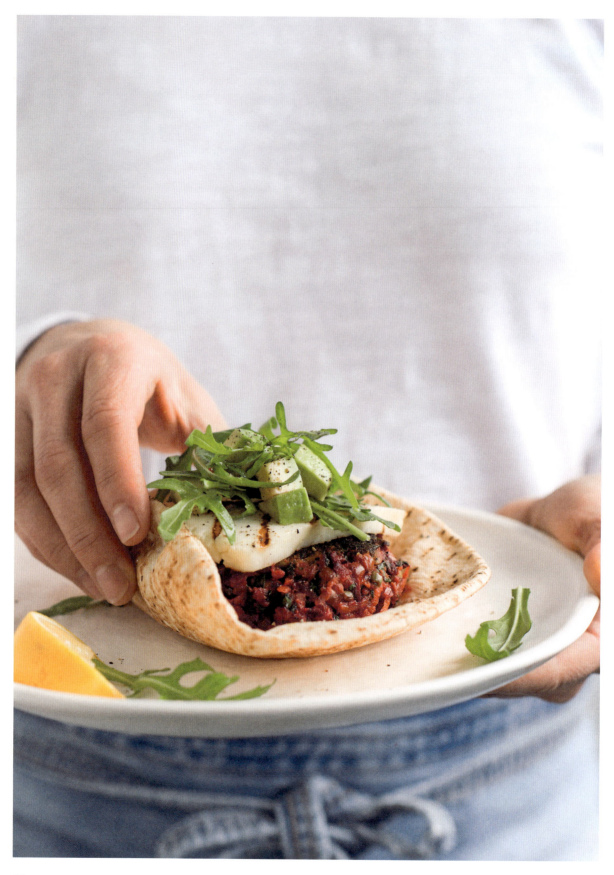

VEGIE BURGERS

PREP TIME: **30 MINUTES** COOK TIME: **10 MINUTES**

These burgers have a lot of ingredients, but most of them will already be in your pantry, and it really won't matter if you're missing a spice or two. You can serve the patties in a wholemeal bun with your choice of extras, or simply with a salad.

MAKES 6 PATTIES

- ¾ cup (145 g) tinned chickpeas, rinsed
- 1 garlic clove, roughly chopped
- 1 tablespoon flat-leaf parsley leaves
- ½ teaspoon ground turmeric
- ½ teaspoon ground cumin
- ½ teaspoon ground coriander
- ½ teaspoon garam masala
- ¼ teaspoon chilli flakes
- 1 cup (125 g) grated pumpkin
- ½ cup (70 g) grated beetroot
- ¼ cup (35 g) finely diced celery
- 4 spring onions, finely chopped
- ½ cup (110 g) tinned lentils, rinsed
- ½ cup mint leaves, finely chopped
- 2 tablespoons coriander leaves, chopped
- 2 tablespoons grated parmesan cheese
- 20 g pepitas (pumpkin seeds), roughly chopped
- 2 large eggs, lightly whisked
- 1 tablespoon lemon juice
- 1 teaspoon freshly ground black pepper
- 1 teaspoon salt
- 1 tablespoon extra virgin olive oil

Combine the chickpeas, garlic, parsley and spices in a food processor. Process in short bursts until the mixture is smooth.

Transfer the chickpea mixture to a large bowl and add all of the remaining ingredients, except the oil, then mix until well combined. Squeeze handfuls of the mixture to remove the excess liquid.

Shape the mixture into six patties. Refrigerate until needed.

Heat the oil on a barbecue hotplate or in a large frying pan over medium heat. Gently fry the patties for 3–4 minutes on each side or until browned and cooked through.

TIPS

→ These patties freeze well and can also be refrigerated for up to 5 days. Once you have browned the patties on each side, you can set them aside until required, then reheat in a 180°C oven for 5 minutes.
→ Serve the patties in a wholemeal pita bread or bun and add your choice of extras, such as grilled haloumi, avocado, rocket, baby spinach, sauerkraut, kimchi, egg, beetroot, tomato salsa or a yoghurt dressing.

nutrition per pattie Energy **540kJ** ‖ Protein **9g** ‖ Fat **5g** (Sat Fat 1g, Poly 1g, Mono 2g)
Carbohydrate **10g** ‖ Fibre **4g**
(without accompaniments)

BEEF, BEET AND ZUCCHINI BURGERS

PREP TIME: **15 MINUTES, PLUS 30 MINUTES CHILLING** COOK TIME: **10 MINUTES**

Our families absolutely love these burgers and the added vegies not only give a serious nutritional boost, they add moisture and flavour to the patties. We have used a combination of beef and pork mince, but you could use just one type or substitute any other meat. Serve the burgers in a bun with any combination of accompaniments or simply serve them with oven-baked chips and a lovely big salad.

MAKES 12 PATTIES

500 g beef mince

500 g pork mince

1 large beetroot, grated

2 small zucchini, grated

1 onion, grated

⅓ cup flat-leaf parsley leaves, finely chopped

1 cup (60 g) fresh wholegrain breadcrumbs

1 egg

2 tablespoons Worcestershire sauce

1 tablespoon dijon mustard

1 tablespoon wholegrain mustard

Add all of the ingredients to a large bowl and season with salt and freshly ground black pepper. Mix with your hands until well combined.

Divide the mixture into 12 patties. Freeze half of the patties for another meal. Put the remaining patties on a plate and refrigerate for 30 minutes or until firm.

Heat a barbecue hotplate or a frying pan to medium and cook the patties for about 5 minutes on each side or until done to your liking.

TIPS

→ Make your own wholegrain breadcrumbs by blitzing sliced bread in a powerful blender or food processor until fine. This works best with bread that's a couple of days old.

→ Serve the patties in a wholegrain or wholemeal burger bun with your choice of extras, such as lettuce, tomato, cucumber, beetroot, cheddar cheese, grilled haloumi cheese, fried egg, hummus, caramelised onion relish, tomato relish, tomato sauce, barbecue sauce or Mint Yoghurt (page 117).

→ Add any left-over cooked burger patties to wraps spread with hummus and topped with salad for school lunchboxes.

nutrition per pattie Energy **590kJ** ‖ Protein **20g** ‖ Fat **5g** (Sat Fat 2g, Poly 1g, Mono 2g)
Carbohydrate **5g** ‖ Fibre **1g**
(without accompaniments)

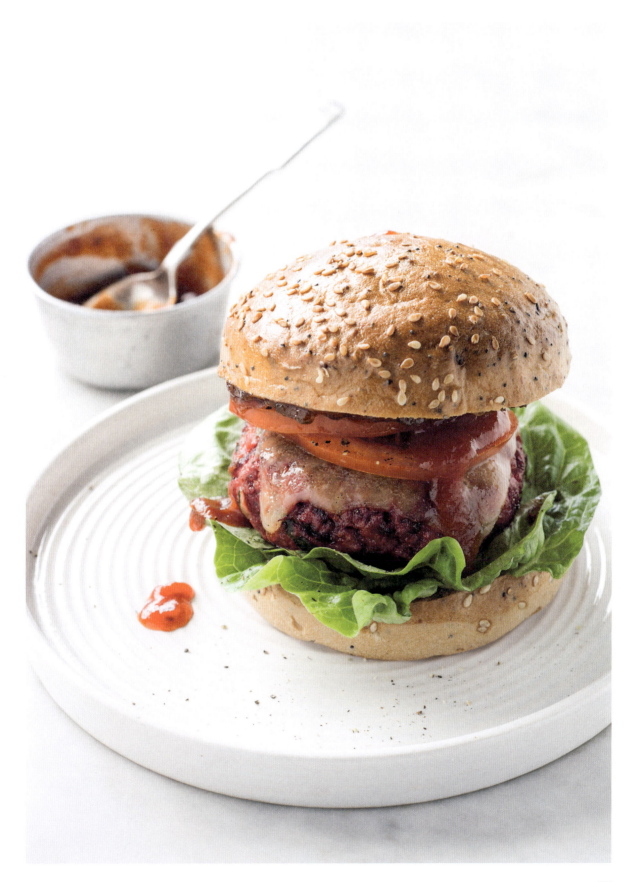

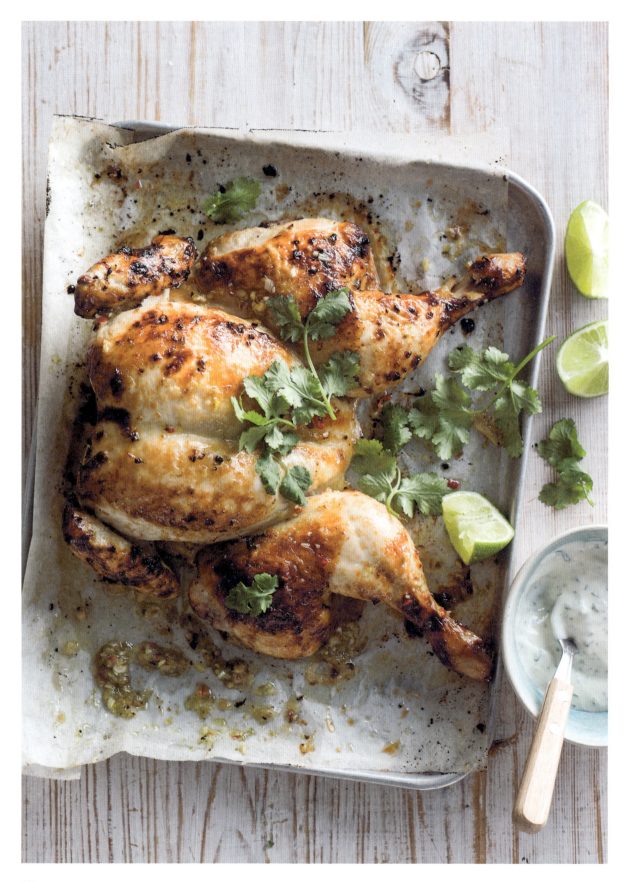

BARBECUED CHILLI LIME CHICKEN

PREP TIME: **10 MINUTES, PLUS 1 HOUR MARINATING** COOK TIME: **1 HOUR**

Chicken cooked on the bone tends to be much tastier and it's also usually cheaper to buy a whole bird rather than individual cuts. To cut down on time, get the chicken marinating the night before or in the morning, so that it's ready to throw onto the barbecue (or into the oven, if you prefer) that evening.

SERVES 4

2 tablespoons extra virgin olive oil
Grated zest and juice of 2 limes
¼ cup finely chopped coriander
   roots
2 tablespoons honey
2 garlic cloves, crushed
1 bird's eye chilli, seeded and
   finely chopped
1 teaspoon freshly ground
   black pepper
1.2–1.4 kg free-range chicken,
   butterflied

YOGHURT DRESSING
1 cup (260 g) Greek-style yoghurt
Grated zest and juice of ½ lime
1 tablespoon coriander leaves,
   chopped

Whisk the oil, lime zest and juice, coriander root, honey, garlic, chilli and pepper in a bowl until combined.

Put the butterflied chicken in a large glass dish and pour in the marinade. Turn the chicken to coat with the marinade. Marinate in the fridge for at least 1 hour, preferably longer.

Heat a barbecue grill to high, then reduce the heat to medium. Drain the chicken from the marinade and place over indirect heat, skin side up. Close the lid of the barbecue and cook for 30 minutes. Turn the chicken over, close the lid again and cook for another 30 minutes or until the chicken is completely cooked through.

To make the yoghurt dressing, combine the yoghurt, lime zest, lime juice and chopped coriander. Season with freshly ground black pepper.

Serve the whole barbecued chicken as a shared platter or cut the chicken into pieces and serve with the yoghurt dressing and homemade oven-baked or air-fried chips and salad.

TIPS

→ You can also cook the chicken in an oven that's been preheated to 180°C.
→ Use the marinade for any cut of chicken or for chicken skewers.

nutrition per serve   Energy **1420kJ** ‖ Protein **34g** ‖ Fat **14g** (Sat Fat 3g, Poly 1g, Mono 8g)
Carbohydrate **18g** ‖ Fibre **3g**
(with 100g cooked chicken)

A VEGO IN THE FAMILY

While we encourage everyone to embrace more plant foods, what do you do if a family member wants to cut out some or all animal foods? Have a chat about their reasoning for cutting out animal foods – is it for ethical or perceived health reasons?

Try to understand their point of view and ensure they have correct information, and establish what foods they wish to avoid. Do they want to cut out red meat? Are they happy to continue to eat eggs and dairy but avoid all animal flesh? Are they happy to continue eating seafood? Or do they want to be strictly vegan?

The more foods that are avoided, the harder it becomes to meet nutrient requirements, particularly for younger kids and teenagers who are growing and developing. Below are the key nutrients found in animal foods and suggestions for alternative foods you could introduce to replace them.

Protein

We think of protein as coming from meat, fish, eggs and dairy products, but there are also plenty of plant foods that supply protein. In fact, we can all benefit from replacing some animal protein with plant protein.

Only a few plant foods, such as soy and quinoa, contain all the essential amino acids. These are the amino acids that we cannot make in the body and therefore have to obtain from our diet. Fortunately, plants tend to complement each other and where one is low in or lacking an essential amino acid, another provides it. Provided you include a good variety of plant foods from wholegrains, legumes, nuts and seeds, you will amply meet protein requirements.

The plant foods with the highest levels of protein include:
- → soya beans (and edamame, which are young green soya beans) and foods made from them, such as tofu and tempeh
- → other legumes such as chickpeas (and hummus), red kidney beans, black beans, borlotti beans, cannellini beans and lentils
- → all types of nuts, including peanuts and nut butters
- → seeds, especially chia and hemp, which provide all essential amino acids
- → wholegrains and pseudo-grains including oats, wholemeal pasta and bread, quinoa, amaranth, buckwheat, millet and teff
- → mycoprotein (sold as 'Quorn'), which is made from a fungus
- → various plant-based burger, mince and sausage products, most of which are made from protein extracted from peas, beans or soy, along with other plant extracts and fats to replicate the texture and flavour of meat.

Iron

There are two forms of iron in food – haem and non-haem iron. Meat and seafood provide both forms of iron, but eggs and plant foods only contain non-haem iron. This is important because our absorption of haem iron is considerably greater than our absorption of non-haem iron. Vegetarians need to consume a lot more iron to meet their requirements.

Red meat and liver are fantastic sources of haem iron, so if they are avoided, alternatives need to be found. If shellfish is acceptable, this is a brilliant option. Eggs are also good sources of non-haem iron.

The best plant food sources of iron include fortified breakfast cereals, tofu, wholemeal pasta, wholegrain bread, quinoa, beans, lentils, cashews, oats, edamame and green vegies, such as broccoli, kale and brussels sprouts.

You can improve the absorption of non-haem iron by consuming a food high in vitamin C at the same meal.

Calcium

If dairy foods are being avoided, you can get your calcium from fortified soy milk or other plant-based milk (not all are fortified with calcium so you need to read the label), tofu, teff, rocket, edamame, chia seeds, almonds, okra, kale, cabbage, watercress, bok choy, dried figs and cannellini beans.

If seafood is acceptable, shellfish such as oysters, mussels and prawns, and fish where you eat the bones (e.g. sardines) are terrific for boosting calcium.

Omega-3 fats

We need several different omega-3 fats in the body. Some are only found in animal foods, with the major sources being oily fish and seafood. These are the fats that play crucial roles in brain development in children and brain function in adults, as well as being good for joint and heart health.

It's optimal to include food sources of all types of omega-3 fats, so if seafood and animal foods are being avoided, ensure there's a higher intake of plant omega-3s. Good sources include walnuts, chia seeds, hemp seeds, flaxseeds (also called linseeds) and edamame.

Vitamin B$_{12}$

Vitamin B$_{12}$ is essential for making red blood cells, for the nervous system and brain, and in energy metabolism. It only occurs in animal foods, so vegans must either include B$_{12}$-fortified foods or take a supplement. We only require tiny amounts of vitamin B$_{12}$, so vegetarians who consume eggs and dairy are more than likely getting enough.

With a little knowledge and planning, you can ensure any vegetarians or vegans in your family are getting all the nutrients they need.

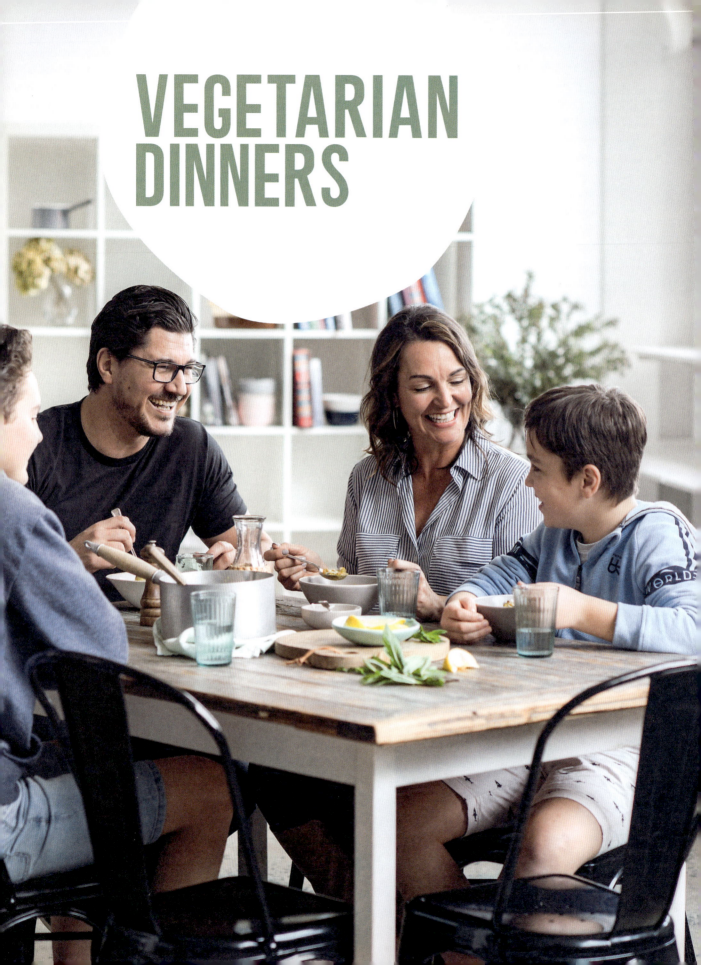

VEGETARIAN DINNERS

MEXICAN SPICED STUFFED CAPSICUMS

PREP TIME: **15 MINUTES** COOK TIME: **45 MINUTES**

Serve these colourful capsicums with a dollop of natural or Greek-style yoghurt (omit the yoghurt for a vegan meal) and a green salad with a drizzle of balsamic vinegar and extra virgin olive oil.

SERVES 4

1 tablespoon extra virgin olive oil

½ red onion, finely diced

150 g sweet potato, finely diced

1 zucchini, finely diced

2 garlic cloves, crushed

200 g firm tofu

400 g tin black beans, drained and rinsed

2 teaspoons ground cumin

1 teaspoon ground coriander

1 teaspoon smoked paprika

1 teaspoon dried oregano

½ teaspoon chilli flakes

1 tablespoon tamari or light soy sauce

40 g almonds, roughly chopped

¼ cup coriander leaves, roughly chopped

4 red capsicums

Preheat the oven to 180°C.

Heat the oil in a large frying pan over medium heat. Sauté the onion until soft and translucent. Add the sweet potato, zucchini and garlic and cook until the sweet potato starts to soften, about 5–6 minutes.

Crumble the tofu and add it to the pan, along with the black beans and spices. Cook, stirring, for 2–3 minutes or until well combined. Stir in the tamari, almonds and coriander, then season with a little salt and freshly ground black pepper. Set aside to cool slightly.

Cut a hole in the top of each capsicum large enough to spoon in the filling. Reserve the capsicum lids. Cut away any seeds and white membrane inside the capsicums and under the lids.

Spoon the filling into the capsicums, sit them upright on a baking tray or in an ovenproof dish and top with the lids. Bake for 30 minutes or until the capsicums are softened and slightly wrinkled. Serve warm.

TIP

→ You can prepare the stuffed capsicums in advance and store them in the fridge for up to 2 days, ready to bake.

nutrition per serve   Energy **1460kJ** Protein **19g** Fat **16g** (Sat Fat 2g, Poly 4g, Mono 8g) Carbohydrate **30g** Fibre **14g**

GADO GADO VEGETABLES WITH TEMPEH

PREP TIME: **20 MINUTES** 🍳 COOK TIME: **20 MINUTES**

Tempeh is a traditional fermented Indonesian food made from soya beans. Because the whole bean is used, it retains more of the vitamins, minerals, protein and fibre than tofu. It's a terrific source of protein for vegans and vegetarians.

SERVES 4

100 g tempeh, cut into 2 cm cubes

2 tablespoons hoisin sauce
(page 105 or store-bought)

280 g sweet potato, cut into
chunks

2 eggs

½ Chinese cabbage, sliced

1 large carrot, halved lengthways
and diagonally sliced

125 g green beans, ends trimmed,
halved

125 g fresh or tinned baby corn,
halved lengthways

2 cups (110 g) English spinach,
roughly chopped

1¼ cups (145 g) bean sprouts

1 tablespoon extra virgin olive oil

4 baby cucumbers or 1 Lebanese
cucumber, cut into chunks

1 small handful Thai basil leaves

1 small handful mint leaves

1 tablespoon crushed roasted
peanuts

¼ cup (60 ml) Hoisin Dressing
(page 105)

1 lime, cut into wedges

Put the tempeh in a small bowl and add the hoisin sauce. Leave to marinate for at least 15 minutes while you prepare the vegetables.

Bring a large saucepan of lightly salted water to the boil. Add the sweet potato and eggs and boil for 8 minutes, then remove the eggs and set aside to cool. Check the sweet potato and continue cooking until tender, then scoop from the water using a sieve or slotted spoon.

Add the cabbage, carrot, beans and corn to the pan of boiling water. Cook for 2–3 minutes or until tender, then scoop the vegetables out of the water and set aside.

Blanch the spinach and the bean sprouts in the boiling water for 30 seconds, taking care not to overcook them. Strain and set aside.

Heat the oil in a frying pan over medium heat. Add the drained tempeh and gently fry, turning, until browned all over. (Do not add any excess marinade to the pan as it will burn.)

Peel the boiled eggs and cut in half.

Arrange all of the vegetables on a large platter, together with the tempeh and boiled eggs. Scatter the herbs over the salad and sprinkle with the peanuts. Spoon the hoisin dressing over the top. Serve with lime wedges.

nutrition per serve   Energy **1830kJ** ‖ Protein **20g** ‖ Fat **25g** (Sat Fat 4g, Poly 7g, Mono 12g)
Carbohydrate **27g** ‖ Fibre **12g**

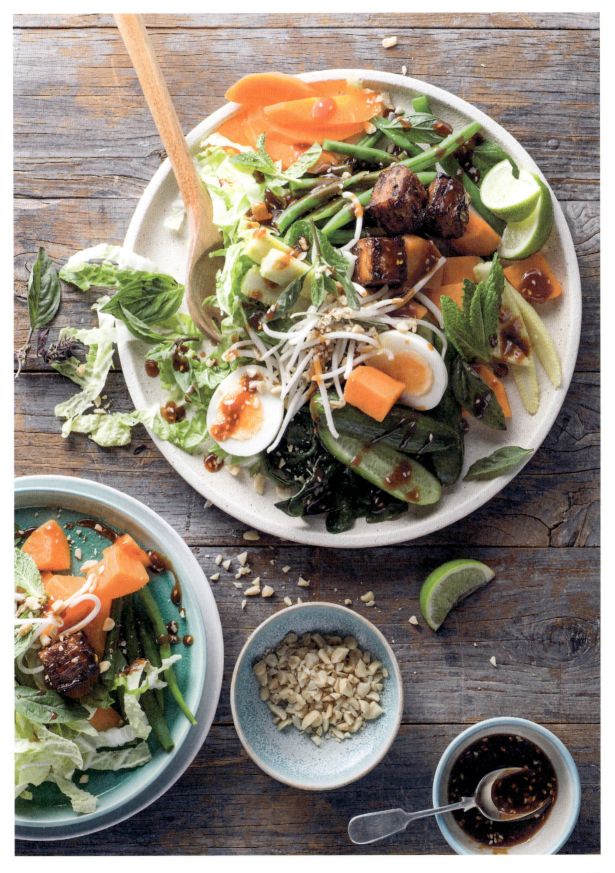

BROCCOLI KALE PESTO AND MOZZARELLA TOASTIE

PREP TIME: 10 MINUTES 🍞 **COOK TIME: 5 MINUTES**

We have given the good old cheese toastie a nutrient boost. Making a pesto is a great way to add flavour as well as nutrition. Make more than you need and store it in a jar in the fridge for up to a week. Pouring a little extra virgin olive oil over the top of the jar will seal out the air and help to preserve the bright green colour.

SERVES 4

- 2 cups (120 g) broccoli florets
- 30 g kale, stems removed, roughly chopped
- ½ cup (40 g) grated parmesan cheese
- Grated zest of 1 lemon
- 1 tablespoon basil leaves
- 1 tablespoon mint leaves
- ½ teaspoon salt
- ½ teaspoon freshly ground black pepper
- 1 celery stalk, finely chopped
- ¼ cup (30 g) walnuts, finely chopped
- ¼ teaspoon chilli flakes (optional)
- 8 slices wholegrain or rye sourdough
- 120 g mozzarella cheese, grated

Put the broccoli in a microwave-safe bowl with a splash of water and cook on High for 2 minutes. Immediately rinse under cold water to stop the cooking process and to retain the bright green colour. Drain and allow to cool.

Put the broccoli in a food processor with the kale, parmesan, lemon zest, basil and mint. Process in short bursts until the mixture forms a coarse paste. Season the pesto with the salt and pepper.

Transfer the broccoli mixture to a bowl and stir in the celery, walnuts and chilli, if using.

Spread half of the sourdough slices with the broccoli pesto. Top with the grated mozzarella and the remaining bread slices.

Cook the sandwiches in a sandwich press or jaffle maker until the cheese is melted and the bread is crunchy and golden.

TIP

→ You can use sliced bocconcini balls in place of the mozzarella if you wish.

nutrition per serve   Energy **1560kJ** ‖ Protein **22g** ‖ Fat **18g** (Sat Fat 7g, Poly 6g, Mono 4g)
Carbohydrate **26g** ‖ Fibre **7g**

PESTO TOFU SCRAMBLE

PREP TIME: 10 MINUTES **COOK TIME: 5 MINUTES**

Serve this as a pasta sauce or simply with toasted wholemeal sourdough bread. You won't need the whole quantity of pesto for this recipe – transfer the left-over pesto to a jar and store it in the fridge for up to a week.

SERVES 2

1 tablespoon extra virgin olive oil
100 g mushrooms, sliced
250 g firm tofu, crumbled
120 g cherry tomatoes, halved
2 cups (100 g) baby spinach

WALNUT, BASIL AND SPINACH PESTO

10 g sun-dried tomatoes
⅓ cup (45 g) walnuts
20 g parmesan cheese
⅓ cup tightly packed basil leaves
⅔ cup (30 g) baby spinach
1 tablespoon extra virgin olive oil
½ teaspoon freshly ground
   black pepper
½ teaspoon salt

To make the pesto, combine the ingredients in a blender or food processor and process in short bursts until the mixture forms a paste. If the pesto is too thick, add 1 tablespoon water, scrape down the side of the blender and process again.

Heat the oil in a frying pan over medium heat. Sauté the mushrooms for 2 minutes. Add the crumbled tofu, tomatoes and 4 tablespoons of the pesto and stir to combine. Stir in the spinach and cook until wilted. Serve immediately.

TIPS

→ Tofu is one of the best foods to include in a vegetarian menu plan as it is high in protein and calcium.
→ Use the left-over walnut pesto in salad dressings, as a pasta sauce, spread on toast or in a sandwich, or spooned over poached eggs.

nutrition per serve   Energy **1600kJ** ‖ Protein **21g** ‖ Fat **30g** (Sat Fat 4g, Poly 12g, Mono 11g)
Carbohydrate **3g** ‖ Fibre **10g**

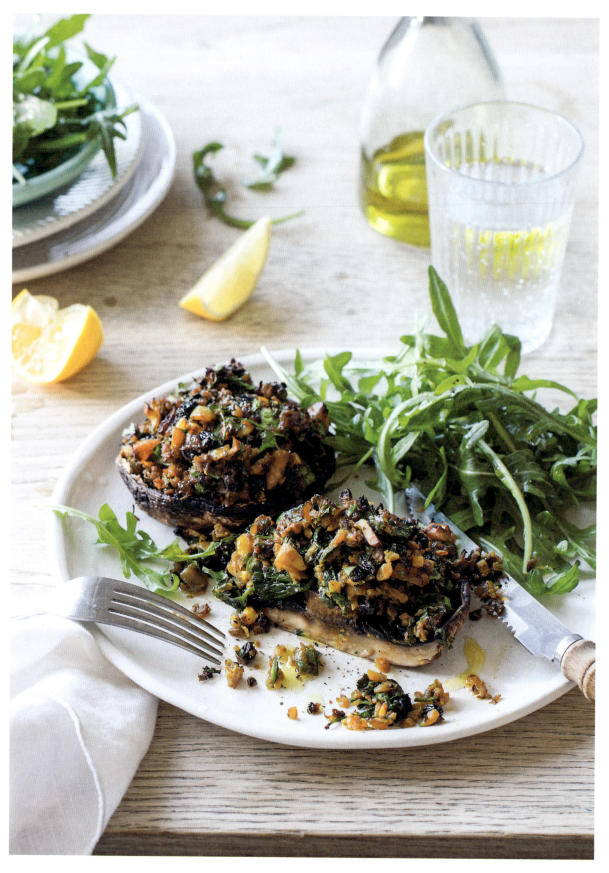

STUFFED FIELD MUSHROOMS WITH SPICED CAULIFLOWER RICE

PREP TIME: 25 MINUTES   **COOK TIME: 40 MINUTES**

These mushrooms are lovely as they are, or for a more substantial meal you can dollop a tablespoon of fresh ricotta cheese or labneh on top of each one, along with a large handful of rocket leaves. Drizzle a little more extra virgin olive oil over the top of the mushrooms and finish with a squeeze of lemon juice.

SERVES 4

8 field mushrooms
500 g cauliflower, roughly chopped
2 tablespoons extra virgin olive oil
1 onion, finely chopped
1 garlic clove, crushed
¼ cup (35 g) cashews, chopped
¼ cup (40 g) currants
2 teaspoons curry powder
1 teaspoon ground turmeric
½ teaspoon smoked paprika
1 tablespoon tamari or light
    soy sauce
2 cups (100 g) baby spinach
½ cup coriander leaves,
    roughly chopped
½ cup flat-leaf parsley leaves,
    roughly chopped
¼ cup mint leaves, chopped
1 teaspoon grated lemon zest
¼ teaspoon salt
½ teaspoon freshly ground
    black pepper

Preheat the oven to 180°C.

Finely dice the mushroom stems and set aside.

Put the cauliflower in a food processor and process in short bursts for a few seconds until it has a rice-like texture.

Heat 1 tablespoon of the oil in a large frying pan over medium heat. Sauté the onion, garlic and chopped mushroom stems until soft. Add the cauliflower, cashews, currants and spices. Cook, stirring, for 5 minutes.

Pour in the tamari, then toss in the spinach, herbs and lemon zest. Season with the salt and pepper.

Fill each mushroom with the cauliflower rice, pressing firmly into a mound. Drizzle the remaining oil over the mushrooms and bake for 30 minutes or until softened and golden. Serve hot or cold.

TIP

→ Don't overprocess the cauliflower or it will turn to mush – just process it in split-second bursts.

nutrition per serve   Energy **1220kJ** ‖ Protein **14g** ‖ Fat **16g** (Sat Fat 2g, Poly 2g, Mono 9g)
Carbohydrate **14g** ‖ Fibre **13g**

KALE, HERB AND GOAT'S CHEESE TART

PREP TIME: **20 MINUTES, PLUS CHILLING** COOK TIME: **50 MINUTES**

SERVES 6

CRUST
¾ cup (95 g) grated beetroot
⅔ cup (70 g) rolled oats
1 cup (150 g) wholemeal plain flour,
  plus extra for dusting
½ teaspoon salt
½ cup (125 ml) extra virgin olive oil

CARAMELISED ONION
2 teaspoons extra virgin olive oil
1 red onion, thinly sliced
2 thyme sprigs, leaves removed
¼ teaspoon salt
2 tablespoons balsamic vinegar

FILLING
2 teaspoons extra virgin olive oil
1 cup (50 g) chopped kale leaves
1 cup (50 g) baby spinach
½ lemon
2 tablespoons flat-leaf parsley
  leaves, finely chopped
2 tablespoons mint leaves,
  finely chopped
1 tablespoon dill, roughly chopped
100 g soft goat's cheese
6 large eggs
300 ml milk
2 tablespoons grated parmesan
  cheese
1 teaspoon ground black pepper

To make the crust, blitz the beetroot, oats, flour and salt in a food processor until it resembles coarse sand. Slowly add the oil and process until the dough just comes together into a ball. Scoop the dough out onto a floured work surface and bring it together with your hands to form a smooth log shape. Roll in plastic wrap and chill in the fridge for at least 1 hour.

Carefully slice the dough lengthways into 5 mm slices. Place the slices in and around the base and sides of a 24 cm tart tin, just fitting them together. Press and smooth the pastry with the back of a spoon, patching and covering any holes. Ensure it is level the whole way around the tin. Place in the freezer for 15–20 minutes to rest. Preheat the oven to 170°C.

Bake the tart case for 20 minutes or until slightly firm to the touch, slightly dry and lighter in colour. Set aside to cool.

While the pastry is cooking, make the caramelised onion. Heat the oil in a frying pan over medium heat. Sauté the red onion, thyme and salt, stirring occasionally, for 10 minutes. Add the vinegar and 1 tablespoon water and cook for 5–10 minutes or until the onion is sticky and darkened in colour. Set aside.

To make the filling, heat the oil in a frying pan over medium–high heat. Sauté the kale and spinach for 2–3 minutes until wilted. Squeeze the lemon juice over the kale mixture and stir in the herbs. Spread the kale mixture over the tart base. Dollop the goat's cheese on top and spread 1–2 tablespoons of the caramelised onion over the goat's cheese. Whisk the eggs, milk and parmesan and season with the black pepper. Pour the egg mixture over the filling.

Bake the tart for 25–30 minutes or until the middle is just set.

nutrition per serve   Energy **2160kJ** ‖ Protein **18g** ‖ Fat **33g** (Sat Fat 8g, Poly 3g, Mono 19g)
Carbohydrate **28g** ‖ Fibre **6g**

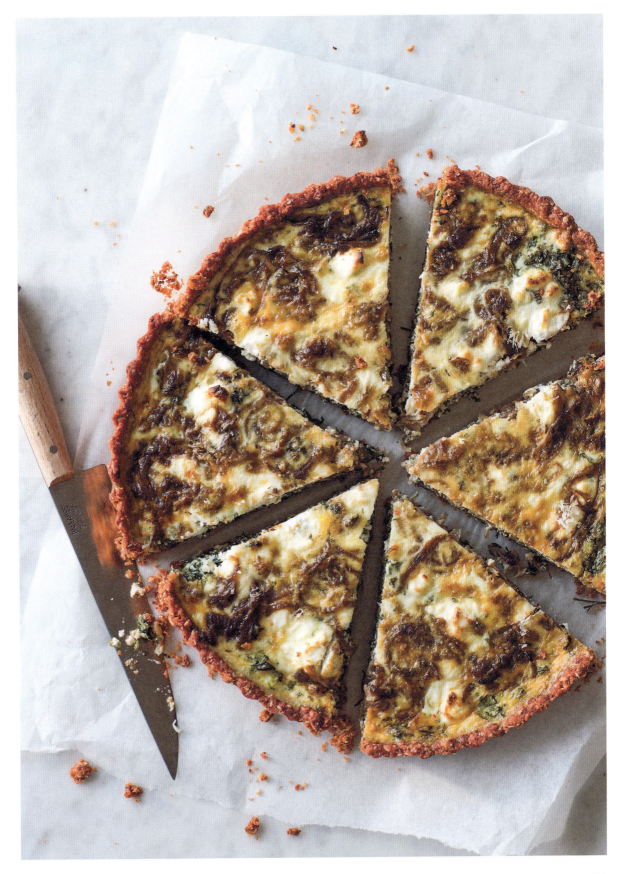

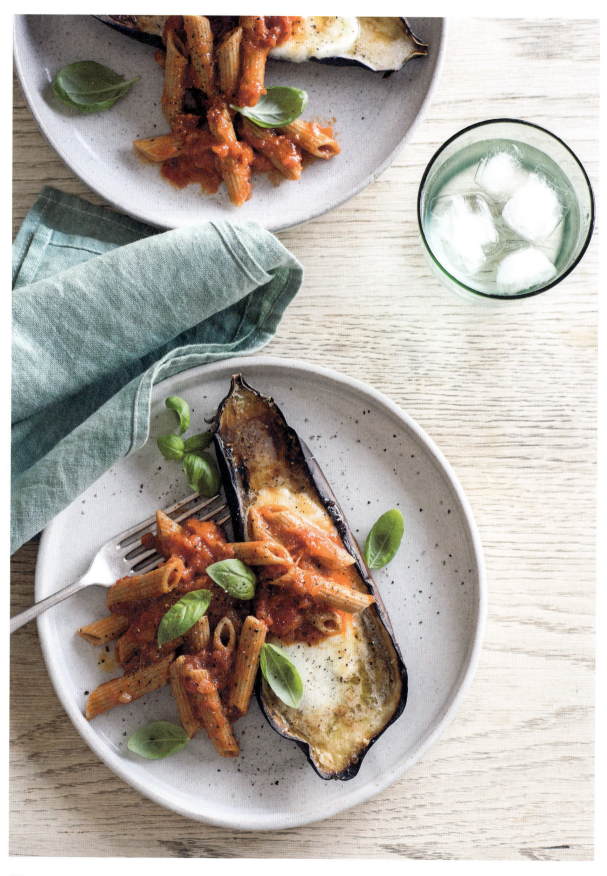

SLOW-COOKED TOMATO RAGU WITH BAKED EGGPLANT AND MOZZARELLA

PREP TIME: 15 MINUTES · **COOK TIME: 1 HOUR 10 MINUTES**

Enjoy this delicious pasta with a green salad or sautéed spinach leaves sprinkled with lemon juice, extra virgin olive oil and freshly ground black pepper.

SERVES 4

1½ tablespoons extra virgin olive oil

1 large brown onion, finely diced

1 garlic clove, crushed

1½ teaspoons salt

2 x 400 g tins Italian tomatoes

4 basil leaves, roughly chopped, plus extra leaves to serve

2 small eggplant

260 g wholemeal penne or macaroni pasta

120 g buffalo mozzarella, cut into 8 slices

2 tablespoons grated parmesan cheese

Heat 1 tablespoon of the oil in a saucepan over medium–low heat. Add the onion, garlic and a pinch of the salt and sauté for 4–5 minutes or until the onion is soft and translucent. Pour in the tomatoes and crush them using the back of a wooden spoon. Reduce the heat to a simmer and cook for 1 hour, stirring occasionally and crushing the tomatoes as you stir. The ragu will thicken and darken when it's ready. Season to taste and add the basil.

Halfway through the ragu cooking time, prepare the eggplant. Preheat the oven to 180°C. Line a baking tray with baking paper. Cut the eggplant in half lengthways and place on the tray, cut side up. Drizzle with the remaining 2 teaspoons of oil and sprinkle with a little salt. Bake for 20–30 minutes or until the eggplant is soft and tender.

Meanwhile, bring a large saucepan of water to the boil. Cook the pasta according to the packet instructions until al dente, then drain.

Top each eggplant half with two slices of the mozzarella and a sprinkle of parmesan. Return to the oven on the grill setting and bake until the cheese is melted and golden.

Place an eggplant half on each plate and top with the pasta and ragu. Serve topped with basil leaves.

nutrition per serve Energy **2030kJ** ‖ Protein **21g** ‖ Fat **17g** (Sat Fat 7g, Poly 1g, Mono 7g) Carbohydrate **53g** ‖ Fibre **16g**

DECODING FOOD LABELS

Being able to buy at least some foods in a tin, bottle or packet is a helping hand and a bonus of modern living. The challenge is working out how to use packaged foods, while still feeding ourselves and our families well. The trick to choosing the healthiest options is being able to understand food labels.

Front-of-pack labelling

The front of the pack contains some nutrition information, but there is also marketing glitz and glamour! The marketing and the nutrition content are often badly aligned. For example, a breakfast cereal might boast how many vitamins and minerals it contains (usually added), yet be 30 per cent added sugar, high in refined starch and contain artificial colours or flavourings.

In Australia, the Health Star Rating (HSR) system attempts to give a quick assessment of the healthfulness of products to help you compare foods across the same category, such as breakfast cereals. Stars are awarded on a points basis, with points deducted for the 'negative nutrients' – saturated fat, sodium and sugar – and for kilojoules. Points are gained for 'positive nutrients' from vegies, fruit, nuts and legumes, and for protein and fibre content.

This system is not without its flaws – food and nutrition are complex and not easily assessed by looking at only a few factors. Nevertheless, it's the best system we have to date and it will hopefully continue to improve. Use the star rating as a guide, but don't let it be your only tool, and remember that it's designed only for packaged, multi-ingredient foods.

Back-of-pack labelling

The back of the pack includes the nutrition information panel (NIP) as well as the ingredients list, where you will see exactly what has gone into making the product. The ingredients are listed from greatest to smallest by weight, which means that the first few ingredients are key. A healthy product will generally have a list of ingredients that you recognise as foods, so that you could, in theory (with the recipe), buy the ingredients for yourself and make it at home.

The NIP gives the nutrition data for both 100g of the product and per serve. If you're comparing products, use the 'per 100g' column, as serve sizes often differ. The 'per serve' column is useful for understanding what you are getting in a serve, but first look at how many serves are in the pack.

ENERGY: The average adult requires 8700kJ (2080kcal) a day, although we all require different levels of kilojoules depending on factors such as gender, size and activity level. You don't need to be counting the kilojoules in everything you eat, but having an awareness of what the figures mean can be helpful. As a general guide, snack products should be no more than 750kJ (180kcal), unless you have very high energy needs.

PROTEIN: The NIP will give the grams of protein per serve or per 100g of the product. We can ably meet our protein requirements from whole foods, so adding extracted and refined protein powders to products to boost their protein content is generally unnecessary. Most of us get plenty of protein from whole foods such as meat, seafood, eggs, tofu, beans or yoghurt.

FAT: Values are given for total fat and saturated fat. Some products might also list polyunsaturated and monounsaturated fat. A low-fat food has less than 3g of fat per 100g and a low-fat liquid has less than 1.5g fat per 100g. Low-fat foods may have fewer kilojoules, but they are not always healthy. The quality of the fat is important, so look for products that contain primarily polyunsaturated or monounsaturated fats and low levels of saturated fats. Look at the ingredients list to see what oil is included.

CARBOHYDRATE: There will be a total carbohydrate value as well as an indication of how much of the carbohydrate is sugars. Note that the sugars include both naturally present and added sugars. If the sugar content is more than 15g per 100g, look for how many added sugars there are and how high up they are on the ingredients list. Refined starch is just as bad as added sugar, so also look for maltodextrin, any ingredient with the word 'starch' in it, and flour that is not specified as wholegrain or wholemeal.

FIBRE: Fibre is the group of carbohydrates that we can't break down and which therefore pass into the colon undigested. Some pass straight through and help keep us regular; others are fermented by the resident microbes, supporting a healthy, diverse microbiome. Not all foods list the fibre content, which usually means it is low. To qualify as a 'good' source of fibre, a product must contain 4g of fibre per serve, and 7g per serve for an 'excellent' source of fibre. For breads, look for those with at least 6g of fibre per 2 slices; for breakfast cereals, look for at least 10g per 100g.

SODIUM (SALT): Salt is usually present in foods as sodium chloride and hence is listed as sodium. Foods with less than 400mg sodium per 100g are 'low salt', and those with less than 120mg are 'very low salt'. Bear in mind that your daily total of sodium should be no higher than 2000mg.

Don't get too caught up in numbers and nutrition information panels... if most of your diet is made up of whole foods, balanced using the Plate template (page 81, you're well on your way to a healthy diet.

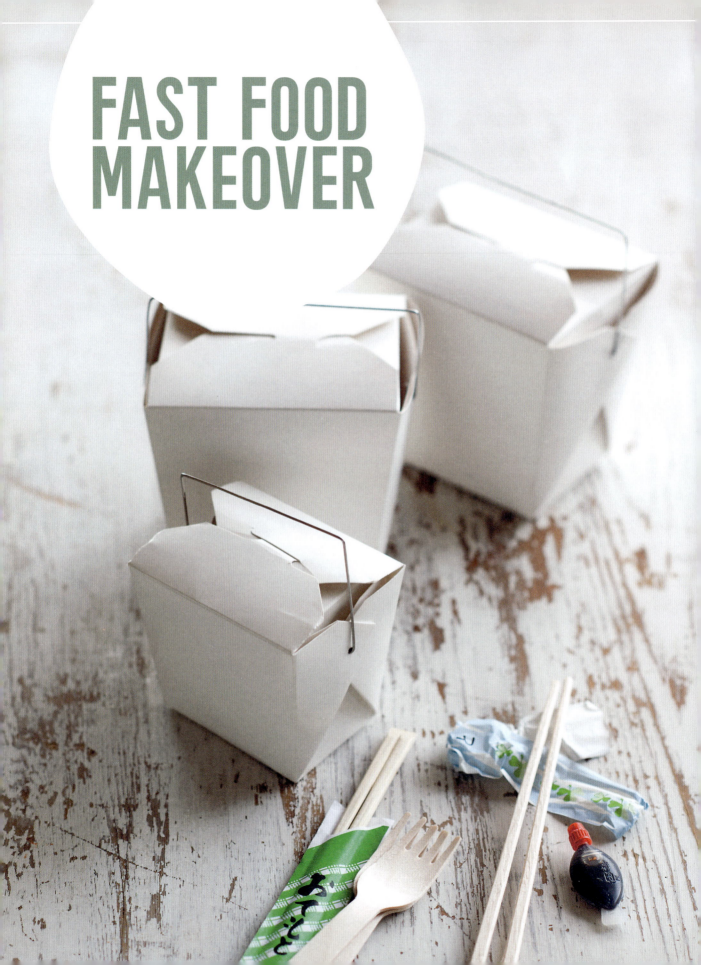

FAST FOOD MAKEOVER

CHICKEN AND PRAWN FRIED RICE

PREP TIME: **10 MINUTES** COOK TIME: **15 MINUTES**

One of the biggest issues with fast food is the cheap, refined oils that are used for cooking. Making your own fried rice at home is so easy and by ensuring you use the most nutritious oil – extra virgin olive oil – you can quickly make a healthy family meal.

SERVES 4

60 g frozen shelled edamame
2 tablespoons extra virgin olive oil
4 large eggs, lightly whisked
2 x 250 g microwavable pouches
    cooked brown rice
3 spring onions, finely chopped
2 cm piece ginger, grated
1 garlic clove, crushed
90 g broccolini, chopped
200 g skinless chicken breast
    fillet, thinly sliced
200 g raw prawns, finely chopped
½ cup (60 g) frozen peas, thawed
1 cup (155 g) finely grated carrot
½ teaspoon ground white pepper
2 tablespoons shaoxing rice wine
    or dry sherry
2 tablespoons oyster sauce

Cook the frozen edamame in a saucepan of boiling water for 2–3 minutes. Drain and set aside.

Heat half the oil in a large frying pan or wok over high heat. When the oil starts to shimmer, add the eggs and cook for 30–45 seconds, gently stirring and folding the outside edges into the centre. Transfer the egg to a plate.

Heat the rice according to the packet instructions. Set aside.

Heat the remaining oil in the same pan over medium heat. Gently sauté the spring onion, ginger and garlic until softened but not coloured. Stir in the broccolini, then add the chicken and sauté for another 2–3 minutes. Add the prawns and stir-fry for 2 minutes or until cooked through.

Stir in the heated rice, then add the edamame, peas, grated carrot, white pepper, rice wine, oyster sauce and the roughly chopped egg. Taste for seasoning and serve immediately.

TIPS

→ You can also use 1 cup (200 g) raw basmati rice, cooked according to the packet instructions.
→ For a vegetarian meal, replace the chicken and prawns with firm tofu or tempeh, replace the oyster sauce with tamari or light soy sauce and add 1 teaspoon sesame oil.

nutrition per serve Energy **2160kJ** ‖ Protein **36g** ‖ Fat **17g** (Sat Fat 3g, Poly 2g, Mono 9g)
Carbohydrate **49g** ‖ Fibre **6g**

LAYERED MEXICAN BEAN DIP

PREP TIME: **15 MINUTES** COOK TIME: **10 MINUTES**

SERVES 6-8

1 cup (260 g) Greek-style yoghurt
Juice of ½ lemon or lime
½ cup (125 ml) tomato salsa
3 radishes, cut into sticks
½ red capsicum, diced
1 Lebanese cucumber, diced
1 green chilli, thinly sliced (optional)
½ cup (50 g) grated cheddar
    cheese

REFRIED BEANS

1 tablespoon extra virgin olive oil
½ brown onion, finely diced
1 small garlic clove, crushed
400 g tin black beans or red kidney
    beans, drained and rinsed
1½ teaspoons ground cumin
1½ teaspoons smoked paprika
½ teaspoon cayenne pepper
½ teaspoon salt

GUACAMOLE

2 ripe avocados
½ garlic clove, crushed
Juice of 1 lemon or lime
¼ cup coriander leaves
1 red chilli, diced, or 2–3 drops of
    Tabasco sauce (optional)
1 teaspoon sesame seeds (optional)

To make the refried beans, heat the oil in a frying pan over medium heat. Gently fry the diced onion and garlic until soft. Add the beans and mash with a fork. Add the cumin, paprika, cayenne pepper and salt and mash to combine. Cook for 2–3 minutes, then stir in ½ cup (125 ml) water to loosen the mixture. Set aside to cool completely.

To make the guacamole, scoop the avocado flesh into a bowl and add the remaining ingredients. Mash everything together until the guacamole is as chunky or smooth as you like. Season with a little salt and freshly ground black pepper.

Whisk the yoghurt and lemon or lime juice together until smooth. Season with freshly ground black pepper.

Mix the tomato salsa with the radishes, capsicum, cucumber and chilli, if using.

To assemble the dip, spread the refried beans over the base of a 30 cm serving dish and sprinkle with the cheese. Spread the guacamole over the cheese, then add a layer of yoghurt. Spoon the salsa over the top of the dip just before serving. Serve with hemp blue or wholegrain corn chips and some carrot, capsicum and cucumber sticks.

TIPS

→ Tinned refried beans are readily available in the supermarket. While they're never as good as homemade, they are certainly convenient if you're in a hurry.
→ Remove the seeds from the chilli for a milder heat.

nutrition per serve (8 serves) Energy **810kJ** ‖ Protein **7g** ‖ Fat **12g** (Sat Fat 3g, Poly 2g, Mono 7g)
Carbohydrate **10g** ‖ Fibre **7g**
(without extra accompaniments)

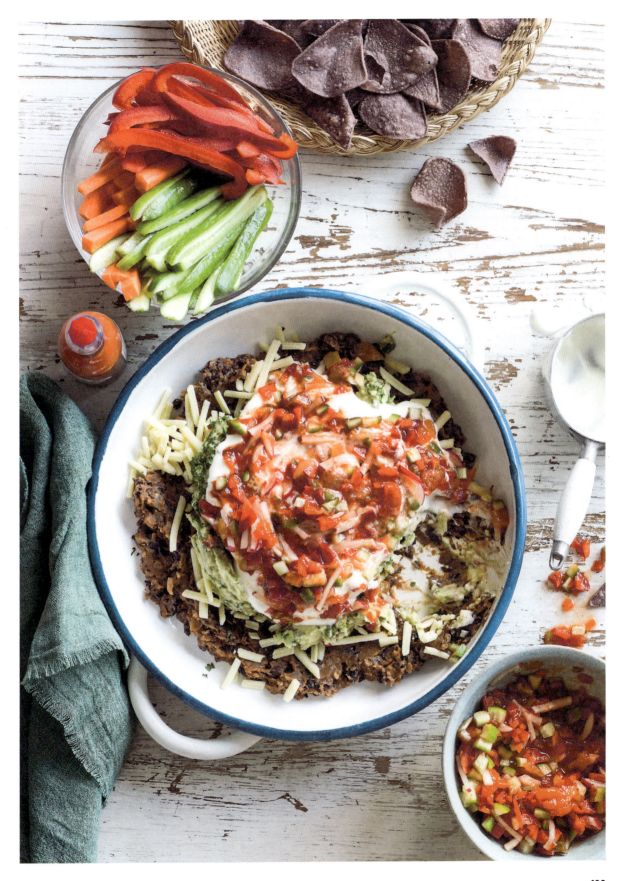

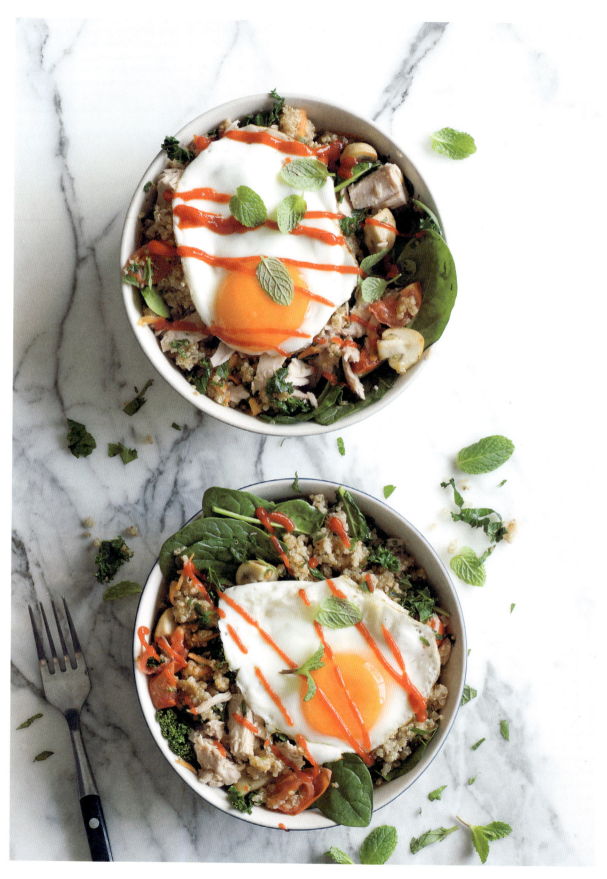

QUINOA NASI GORENG

PREP TIME: **10 MINUTES** COOK TIME: **20 MINUTES**

This is a great go-to lunch or dinner recipe to use up leftovers. It's quick and easy and you can add any lonely ingredient you have in your fridge, freezer or pantry – think corn kernels, peas, capsicum, silverbeet, asparagus, green beans, tinned beans, and even left-over cooked beef, chicken or fish.

SERVES 4

1 cup (200 g) quinoa, rinsed
2 tablespoons extra virgin olive oil
8 button mushrooms, quartered
10 cherry tomatoes, quartered
½ cup (80 g) grated carrot
1 cup (50 g) finely shredded
    kale leaves
2 cups (100 g) baby spinach
1 tablespoon flat-leaf parsley
    leaves, chopped
1 tablespoon mint leaves, chopped,
    plus extra leaves to serve
2 x 185 g tins tuna in springwater
    or extra virgin olive oil, drained
4 large eggs
Hot chilli sauce, such as sriracha,
    to serve (optional)
Lemon wedges, to serve

Put the quinoa in a small saucepan with 1½ cups (375 ml) water and bring to the boil. Reduce the heat, then cover and cook for 12 minutes or until the water has evaporated and the quinoa is light and fluffy. Turn off the heat and stand, covered, for 5 minutes. Using a fork, fluff the quinoa.

Heat 1 tablespoon of the oil in a large frying pan over medium heat. Sauté the mushrooms, tomatoes, carrot and kale until just soft. Stir in the quinoa. Add the spinach, herbs and tuna and stir until everything is well combined and heated through. Remove from the heat and keep warm.

Heat the remaining 1 tablespoon of oil in a frying pan and gently fry the eggs until done to your liking.

Divide the quinoa mixture among four serving bowls and top each with a fried egg. Drizzle with a little chilli sauce, if using, and serve with a wedge of lemon.

nutrition per serve   Energy **1670kJ** ‖ Protein **30g** ‖ Fat **18g** (Sat Fat 3g, Poly 3g, Mono 9g)
Carbohydrate **26g** ‖ Fibre **6g**

BAKED BUFFALO WINGS WITH BLUE CHEESE YOGHURT SAUCE

PREP TIME: 10 MINUTES 🍺 **COOK TIME: 1 HOUR 10 MINUTES**

Footy food at its best! Buffalo wings are a firm favourite, but traditionally they're deep-fried in refined oil and not a healthy choice at all. Our version is baked instead and the result is just as delicious. The spicy sauce does contain butter and maple syrup, but only in small quantities and they are essential for the flavour.

SERVES 6

Extra virgin olive oil, for brushing
18 chicken wings
2 tablespoons baking powder
40 g unsalted butter
¼ cup (60 ml) chilli sauce
2 teaspoons pure maple syrup
4 celery stalks, cut into batons

BLUE CHEESE YOGHURT SAUCE
100 g Gorgonzola or other
   blue cheese
½ cup (130 g) Greek-style yoghurt
Juice of ½ lemon
½ garlic clove, crushed
Pinch of salt
¼ teaspoon freshly ground
   black pepper

To make the blue cheese yoghurt sauce, mash the cheese with a fork, then whisk in the remaining ingredients. Refrigerate until serving time.

Preheat the oven to 140°C. Line a baking tray with foil. Place a wire rack on top of the tray and brush the rack with the oil to help prevent the wings from sticking.

Cut each chicken wing through the joints to create three pieces. Discard the wing tips or reserve them for stock. Pat the wings dry with paper towel, removing as much moisture as possible. Put them in a resealable plastic bag with the baking powder. Seal the bag and shake to coat the wings.

Put the wings on the wire rack, skin side up. Bake on the lower shelf of the oven for 30 minutes. Increase the heat to 220°C and move the tray to the top shelf. Bake for 40 minutes or until the wings are golden and crispy.

Meanwhile, melt the butter in a small saucepan. Whisk in the chilli sauce and maple syrup. Transfer the cooked wings to a large bowl and pour in the spicy sauce, tossing to coat the wings.

Serve the wings with the celery and blue cheese sauce.

nutrition per serve   Energy **1810kJ** ‖ Protein **35g** ‖ Fat **29g** (Sat Fat 12g, Poly 3g, Mono 12g)
Carbohydrate **8g** ‖ Fibre **2g**

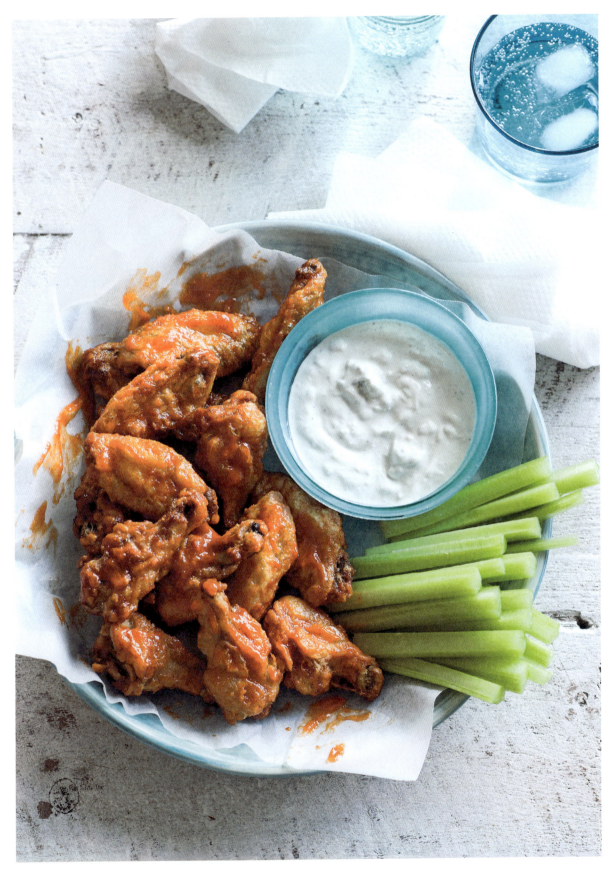

PIZZA

Pizza is pretty much universally loved and although it is thought of as classically Italian, many countries around the world have their own version. It has, of course, veered away from its simple peasant roots, with the addition of all sorts of toppings. We prefer the simplicity of the original, where the emphasis is on a few key quality ingredients such as flavourful tomatoes, fresh basil and good-quality cheese and olives. But you can choose whatever you fancy! Just try not to go overboard as having too many toppings makes it hard to get the base crispy and you'll end up with a soggy pizza. See pages 190–191 for some of our favourite toppings. Make sure you balance the meal with a gorgeous salad.

You can be super-organised and make your bases from scratch using our healthy dough recipe, or take a shortcut and use a bought base. Look for a wholemeal base or use a wholemeal flatbread such as Lebanese or pita bread for a quick meal.

TIPS

→ Pizza dough can be refrigerated for up to 5 days. In fact, seasoned pizza chefs often say the dough is much better if prepared a day in advance. You can also roll out the dough, place it between two sheets of baking paper, then wrap it in foil and freeze it. There is no need to defrost the dough before adding your toppings.
→ Try using lupin flour, lentil flour or any other legume flour in place of besan. You can also substitute a wholegrain gluten-free flour for the wholemeal wheat flour. Experiment to find the flour mix that works best.
→ To make a 'pizza bianco', drizzle a little extra virgin olive oil over the base instead of the tomato sauce and then add your toppings.

PIZZA DOUGH

PREP TIME: **15 MINUTES, PLUS RISING** COOK TIME: **15 MINUTES**

We have nutritionally boosted this pizza dough by using a combination of wholemeal and chickpea flours. This adds plant protein and a range of fibres, including those that fuel healthy gut bugs, and delivers a whole bunch of vitamins, minerals and phytochemicals. It is a little harder to roll out than regular white flour dough – less gluten has the downside of making it less elastic – but it has a deliciously nutty taste. Roll it out nice and thin to achieve a lovely crispy pizza.

MAKES 4 SMALL OR 2 LARGE PIZZAS

2 x 7 g sachets dried yeast
280 ml tepid water
1 tablespoon extra virgin olive oil
1 cup (150 g) wholemeal pizza flour
   (strong, high-protein flour)
1 cup (120 g) besan (chickpea flour)
100 g semolina, plus extra
   for dusting
½ teaspoon salt

Combine the yeast, water and oil in a jug and set aside to activate for 10 minutes. You should see bubbles appear on the surface, which means the yeast is alive and activating.

Using an electric mixer fitted with a dough hook, combine the flours, semolina and salt. Slowly add the activated yeast and water. Knead for 5–10 minutes, or until the dough comes together into a sticky ball. Alternatively, mix the ingredients by hand on a large board.

Sprinkle a little extra semolina over the dough, cover with a damp tea towel and set aside to prove in a warm place for at least 30 minutes or until almost doubled in size.

Preheat the oven to 220°C. Lightly dust a pizza stone or pizza tray with a little semolina.

Knock down the dough and cut it into four balls (or two balls if making larger pizzas). Briefly knead each ball, then roll out to a thickness of about 2 mm.

Place a base on the pizza stone or tray and top with your choice of toppings (see pages 190–191). Bake the pizza for 10–15 minutes or until golden and cooked.

nutrition per base (4 serves) Energy **1530kJ** ‖ Protein **14g** ‖ Fat **7g** (Sat Fat 1g, Poly 2g, Mono 4g)
Carbohydrate **56g** ‖ Fibre **9g**

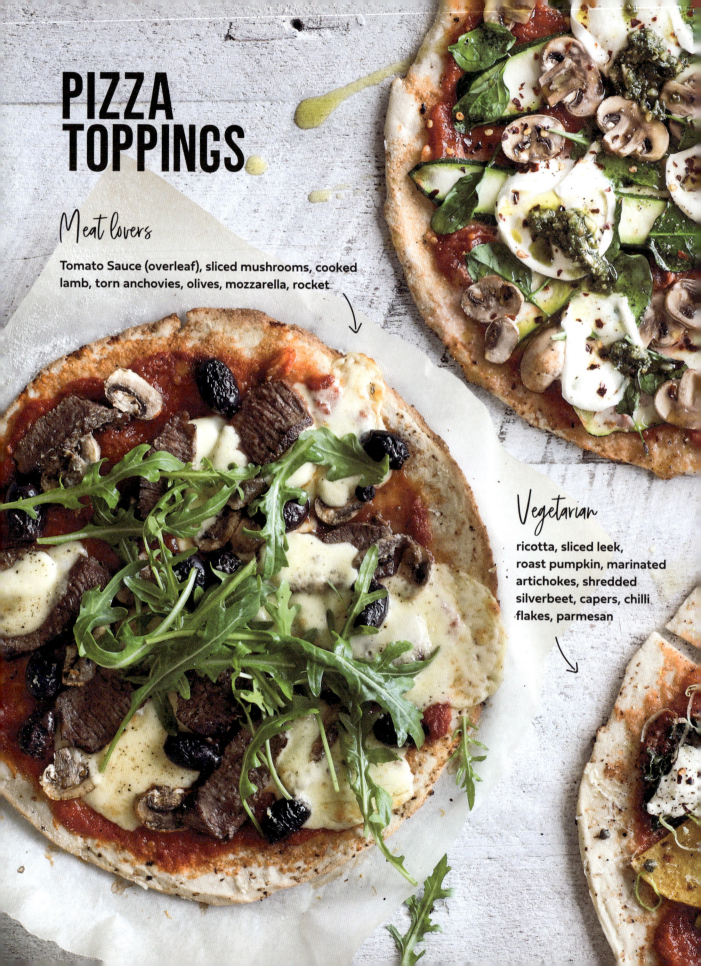

PIZZA TOPPINGS

Meat lovers

Tomato Sauce (overleaf), sliced mushrooms, cooked lamb, torn anchovies, olives, mozzarella, rocket

Vegetarian

ricotta, sliced leek, roast pumpkin, marinated artichokes, shredded silverbeet, capers, chilli flakes, parmesan

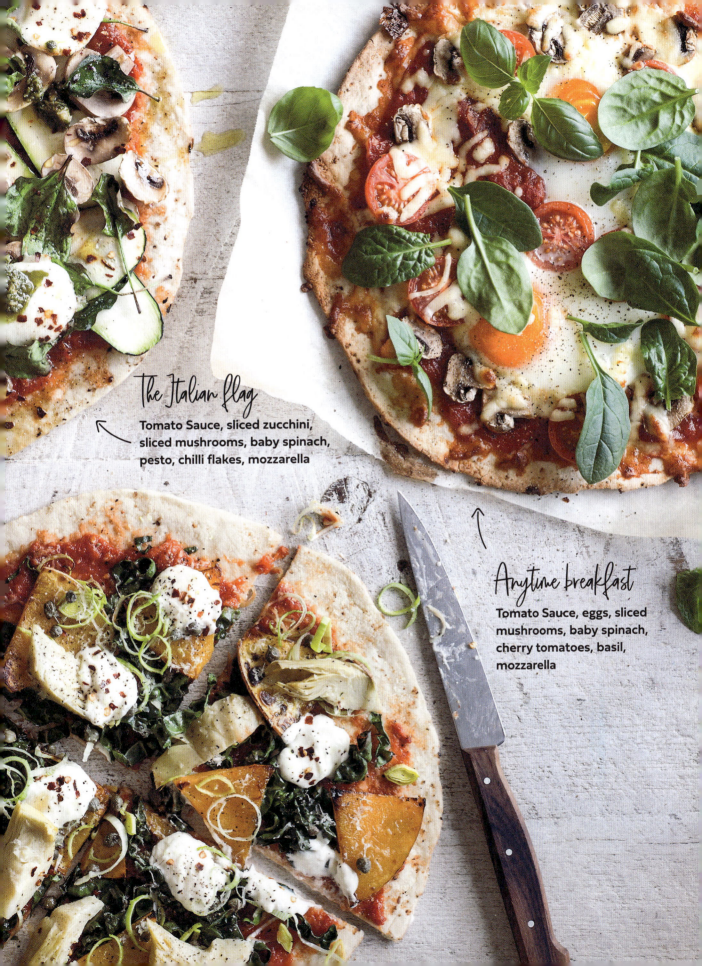

The Italian flag

Tomato Sauce, sliced zucchini, sliced mushrooms, baby spinach, pesto, chilli flakes, mozzarella

Anytime breakfast

Tomato Sauce, eggs, sliced mushrooms, baby spinach, cherry tomatoes, basil, mozzarella

SIMPLE TOMATO SAUCE

PREP TIME: **5 MINUTES** COOK TIME: **15 MINUTES**

This is a versatile sauce that you can use for pizza, pasta or in any recipe where you need a tin of tomatoes with a little more flavour. Stir through some fresh basil leaves at the end for a flavour boost.

SERVES 4

1 garlic clove, peeled
1 tablespoon extra virgin olive oil
½ teaspoon salt
2 x 400 g tins whole tomatoes
½ teaspoon freshly ground
    black pepper

Gently bruise the garlic clove with the side of a knife. Heat the oil in a saucepan over medium heat. Add the garlic, then sprinkle the salt over the garlic. Shake the saucepan and use a wooden spoon to gently press the garlic into the oil. Cook for 2–3 minutes or until the oil is fragrant.

Carefully tip the tomatoes into the pan. Add about ¼ cup (60 ml) water to each tin and swirl to remove the residual tomato juice, then tip into the pan. Cook over medium–low heat for 5–10 minutes, occasionally stirring and crushing any chunks of tomatoes. If the sauce becomes too thick, loosen it with 1–2 tablespoons water.

Season the sauce with the freshly ground black pepper.

TIPS

→ To make this tomato sauce even richer in colour and flavour, finely dice 1 small red or brown onion and add it to the oil along with the garlic. Continue with the basic recipe, but cook at a low simmer with the lid on for about 1 hour to let the flavours develop. The result is a deep, rich and thick sauce that is well worth the wait.

→ Add some salted capers (rinse to remove most of the salt), anchovies (add them to the oil with the onion and they'll melt into the sauce, giving a wonderful depth of flavour), chilli, parsley and/or basil. If you're using dried herbs, add them along with the tomatoes; if you're using fresh herbs, add them at the end of the cooking time.

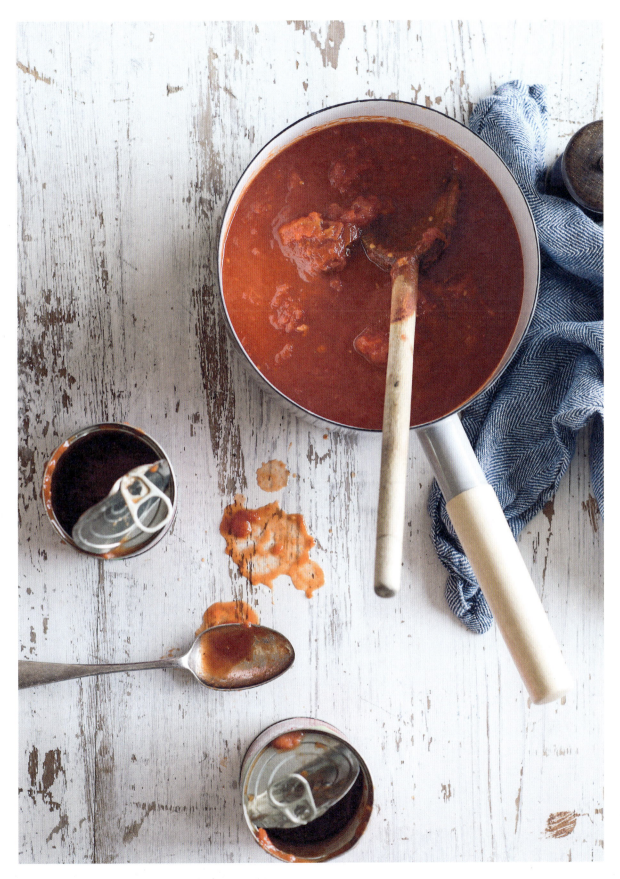

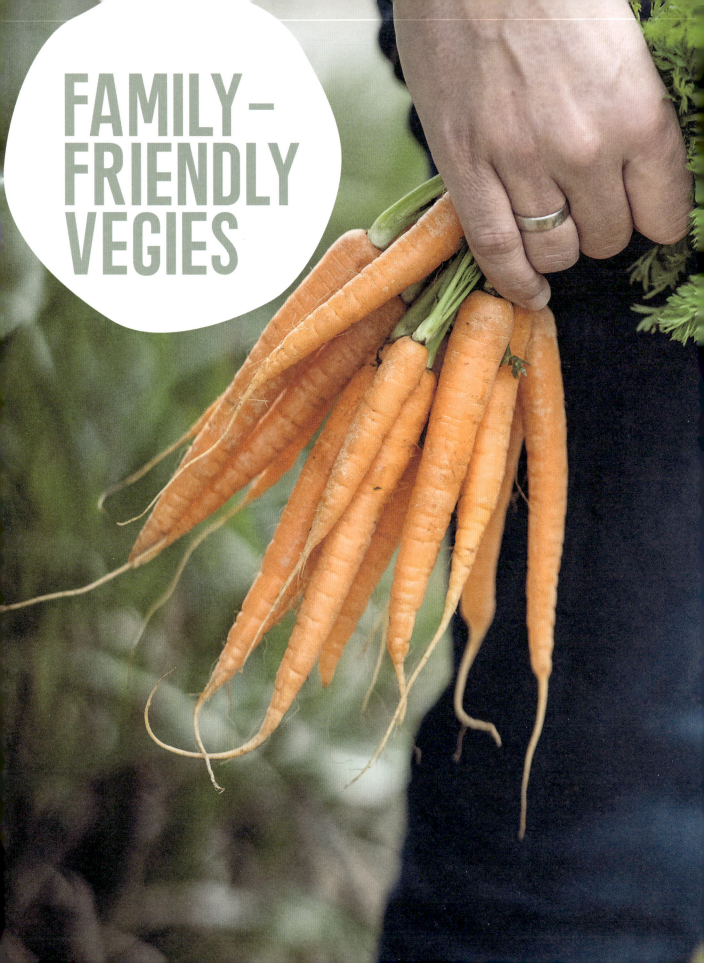

FAMILY-FRIENDLY VEGIES

ROASTED VEGETABLES WITH SRIRACHA TAHINI YOGHURT

PREP TIME: **15 MINUTES** COOK TIME: **30 MINUTES**

This dish is even lovelier if you can get your hands on yellow beetroot when they're in season. They are a little less earthy, but sweet and absolutely beautiful in this dish, which can be served warm or cold.

SERVES 4

1 large golden or red beetroot, peeled and cut into wedges
2 carrots, scrubbed and cut into 4 pieces
2½ cups (310 g) cauliflower florets
1 baby fennel bulb, thickly sliced
1 garlic bulb, skin on, halved horizontally
6 Padrón peppers (see tip)
2 thyme sprigs
1 rosemary sprig
1 tablespoon extra virgin olive oil
½ teaspoon salt
½ teaspoon freshly ground black pepper

SRIRACHA TAHINI YOGHURT

½ cup (130 g) Greek-style yoghurt
⅓ cup (80 ml) lemon juice
½ bunch coriander, leaves and stems finely chopped
2 teaspoons sriracha chilli sauce
1 teaspoon tahini
1 small garlic clove, crushed

Preheat the oven to 180°C. Line a large baking tray with baking paper.

Put the beetroot, carrot and cauliflower in a microwave-safe bowl with a splash of water and cook on High for 5 minutes or until just tender. Transfer the vegetables to the baking tray and add the fennel, garlic, peppers, thyme and rosemary. Drizzle with the oil and season with the salt and pepper.

Roast the vegetables for 20–25 minutes or until golden and tender.

To make the sriracha tahini yoghurt, combine the yoghurt, lemon juice, coriander, chilli sauce, tahini and garlic in a small bowl.

Spread the sriracha tahini yoghurt over a serving plate and top with the roasted vegetables.

TIP

→ Padrón peppers are a Spanish-style chilli pepper, about 5–7 cm long. If they're unavailable, you can simply use a green capsicum instead.

nutrition per serve Energy **730kJ** ‖ Protein **8g** ‖ Fat **7g** (Sat Fat 1g, Poly 1g, Mono 4g)
Carbohydrate **14g** ‖ Fibre **14g**

VEGIE HASH BROWNS

PREP TIME: **15 MINUTES** COOK TIME: **20 MINUTES**

These are delicious as a vegetable side to chicken or meat. You can make large portions, like we have here, to serve as a brunch or lunch meal, or make them a little smaller and serve three or four on the plate.

MAKES 4

2 tablespoons extra virgin olive oil
1 small leek, sliced
2½ cups (310 g) grated sweet potato
3½ cups (280 g) finely shredded Tuscan cabbage or silverbeet
1 tablespoon ground coriander
1 tablespoon ground cumin
2 teaspoons smoked paprika
3 large eggs, lightly whisked
1 teaspoon salt
1 teaspoon freshly ground black pepper
Flat-leaf parsley leaves, to serve
Lemon wedges, to serve

Heat half the oil in a large frying pan over medium–high heat. Sauté the leek for 2 minutes or until softened. Add the sweet potato, Tuscan cabbage, coriander, cumin and paprika and cook until the cabbage has wilted. Transfer the mixture to a large bowl and allow to cool.

Stir the eggs, salt and pepper into the vegetable mixture.

Heat the remaining oil in the same frying pan over medium heat. Cook the hash browns in batches, using a quarter of the mixture for each one, for 2–3 minutes on each side or until golden brown.

Serve the hash browns sprinkled with parsley, with lemon wedges on the side.

TIPS

→ Replace the Tuscan cabbage with silverbeet, English spinach, bok choy or any leafy green vegetable.
→ The hash browns are terrific topped with a poached egg, and vegies such as baby spinach, pea shoots, pan-fried mushrooms, steamed or pan-fried asparagus or brussels sprouts, left-over roasted vegies, fresh or grilled tomatoes, fermented vegies such as sauerkraut or kimchi, or marinated roasted capsicum.
→ You can also add sliced avocado, tomato salsa or relish, beetroot relish or pesto. Sprinkle the hash browns with sesame seeds, pepitas (pumpkin seeds) or sunflower seeds for a little crunch.

nutrition per hash brown

Energy **950kJ** Protein **9g** Fat **14g** (Sat Fat 2g, Poly 1g, Mono 8g)
Carbohydrate **14g** Fibre **6g**

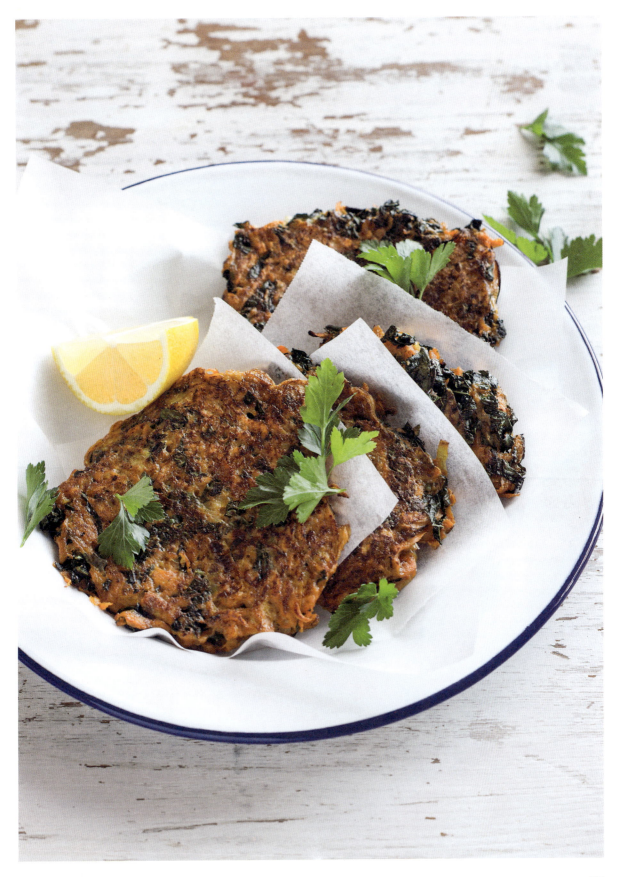

SEMOLINA-CRUSTED SWEET POTATO

PREP TIME: **10 MINUTES**   COOK TIME: **1 HOUR**

You can roast any root vegetable in this way, although the cooking time will vary. The sweet potato is also delicious sprinkled with finely grated parmesan cheese.

SERVES 4–6

1 kg sweet potato, scrubbed and
   cut into large chunks
¼ cup (50 g) semolina
¼ cup (60 ml) extra virgin olive oil
Pinch of salt

Preheat the oven to 200°C.

Put the sweet potato in a large saucepan of water and bring to the boil. Cook for 15 minutes or until you can pierce the sweet potato with a knife. Drain in a colander, then return it to the pan.

Sprinkle the semolina over the sweet potato while shaking the pan. (This will roughen the edges of the sweet potato, resulting in a crispier edge once roasted.)

Pour the oil into a roasting tin. Place the tin in the oven to heat up for about 5 minutes.

Carefully transfer the semolina-covered sweet potato into the hot roasting tin. Bake for 40 minutes, turning once or twice so that each side becomes crisp.

Drain the sweet potato on paper towel to remove any excess oil. Season with the salt and some freshly ground black pepper, then serve immediately.

nutrition per serve (6 serves)   Energy **950kJ** ‖ Protein **4g** ‖ Fat **9g** (Sat Fat 1g, Poly 1g, Mono 7g)
Carbohydrate **29g** ‖ Fibre **5g**

ROASTED BRUSSELS SPROUTS WITH BULGUR AND SOY VINEGAR

PREP TIME: 10 MINUTES, PLUS SOAKING AND MARINATING **COOK TIME: 20 MINUTES**

Give this recipe a shot and rediscover the amazing taste of brussels sprouts. Even if they're not your favourite vegetable, do give them another try. They have a very unfair reputation, but it comes down to how you cook them. Gone are the overboiled, bitter and slightly soggy brussels sprouts of the past!

SERVES 4

¼ cup (45 g) bulgur wheat
2 tablespoons honey
1 tablespoon tamari or light
  soy sauce
1 tablespoon Chinese vinegar
  or brown rice vinegar
1 garlic clove, crushed
½ teaspoon freshly ground
  black pepper
300 g brussels sprouts, halved

Cover the bulgur wheat with 1 cup (250 ml) hot water and leave to soak for 10 minutes, then drain.

Combine the honey, tamari, vinegar, garlic and pepper in a bowl. Add the brussels sprouts and stir to coat. Set aside to marinate for 15 minutes.

Preheat the oven to 200°C. Line a roasting tin or baking tray with baking paper.

Tip the marinated brussels sprouts and half the bulgur wheat into the tin and spread it out. Bake for 20 minutes or until the brussels sprouts are crisp around the edges.

Toss in the remaining bulgur wheat and serve immediately.

TIPS

→ You can replace the bulgur wheat with cooked quinoa.
→ A drizzle of sesame oil over the top and a sprinkle of sesame seeds is a lovely addition. Or squeeze in a little lemon juice for a zingy flavour.

nutrition per serve Energy **500kJ** ‖ Protein **4g** ‖ Fat **<1g** (Sat Fat 0g, Poly 0g, Mono 0g)
Carbohydrate **22g** ‖ Fibre **5g**

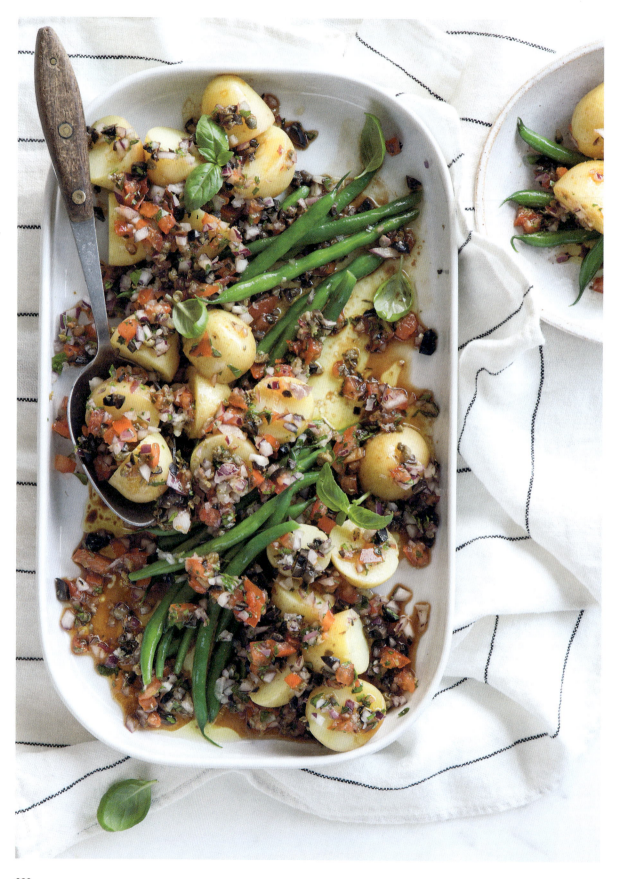

POTATO AND GREEN BEAN SALAD WITH OLIVE CAPER DRESSING

PREP TIME: **20 MINUTES**   COOK TIME: **10 MINUTES**

Combined with the healthy fats of the extra virgin olive oil, this is a superbly healthy and tasty side dish that can be served warm or cold. When you cook and cool potatoes, some of the starch is converted into 'resistant starch'. This cannot be broken down by our own digestive enzymes and it becomes gold-star fuel for the gut microbiome. Always leave the skins on potatoes as this is where most of the fibre is found, along with many of the nutrients and phytochemicals.

SERVES 4

500 g chat potatoes, skin on
140 g green beans, trimmed
1 tablespoon small basil leaves

OLIVE CAPER DRESSING
1 large tomato, seeded and
    finely diced
½ red onion, finely diced
2 tablespoons pitted black olives,
    finely chopped
1 garlic clove, crushed
1 tablespoon salted capers,
    rinsed and chopped
2 tablespoons flat-leaf parsley
    leaves, finely chopped
¼ cup (60 ml) extra virgin olive oil
1 tablespoon white wine vinegar
1 teaspoon balsamic vinegar

To make the dressing, combine the tomato, onion, olives, garlic, capers and parsley in a bowl.

Whisk together the oil and vinegars and season with freshly ground black pepper. Stir the dressing through the tomato mixture and set aside.

Put the potatoes in a large saucepan, cover with water and bring to the boil over high heat. Reduce the heat and simmer for 7–8 minutes or until the potatoes are cooked but not breaking apart. Drain and cut in half.

Steam the green beans for 2 minutes.

Combine the potatoes and beans, and toss with the dressing. Serve warm or cold, topped with the basil leaves.

TIP

→ You can also microwave the potatoes and beans.

nutrition per serve   Energy **1020kJ** ‖ Protein **5g** ‖ Fat **16g** (Sat Fat 2g, Poly 1g, Mono 11g)
Carbohydrate **19g** ‖ Fibre **5g**

PARMESAN CAULI BITES WITH CREAMY CAULI MASH

PREP TIME: **15 MINUTES**   COOK TIME: **30 MINUTES**

You can make these two cauli dishes separately or make them both for a delicious dinner where cauliflower is the hero on the plate. You could serve it with a simple piece of grilled or barbecued meat, fish or tofu, brown or black rice, quinoa or some additional roasted or steamed vegies.

SERVES 4

1 kg cauliflower, cut into bite-sized
    florets
1 tablespoon extra virgin olive oil
½ large onion, diced
1 garlic clove, crushed
¼ teaspoon dried thyme
50 ml milk
½ teaspoon salt
½ teaspoon freshly ground
    black pepper
1 tablespoon flat-leaf parsley
    leaves (optional)
Lemon wedges, to serve

CAULIFLOWER BITES

50 g fresh wholegrain sourdough
    breadcrumbs
1 tablespoon grated parmesan
    cheese
1 tablespoon polenta
2 teaspoons Cajun seasoning
1½ tablespoons cornflour
2 large eggs, lightly whisked
50 ml extra virgin olive oil

Steam the cauliflower for 15 minutes or until tender but not falling apart.

Meanwhile, heat the oil in a frying pan over medium heat. Sauté the onion, garlic and thyme for 4 minutes or until softened but not browned.

Reserve half of the best florets to make the cauliflower bites. Put the remaining cauliflower in a blender with the onion mixture. Blend for 20 seconds. With the motor running, add the milk, salt and pepper and blend for 30 seconds or until smooth. Keep warm while you prepare the cauliflower bites.

To make the cauliflower bites, combine the breadcrumbs, parmesan, polenta and Cajun seasoning in a shallow bowl. Put the cornflour in another shallow bowl. Whisk the eggs in a third shallow bowl. Dust the cauliflower florets in the cornflour, then dip into the egg, turning to coat. Finally, toss the cauliflower in the breadcrumb mixture, covering all over.

Heat the oil in a large frying pan over medium–high heat. Cook the cauliflower in batches, turning, until golden and crisp.

Spread the cauliflower mash on a serving plate and top with the cauliflower bites. Sprinkle with a little parsley, if using, and serve with lemon wedges.

nutrition per serve   Energy **1290kJ** ║ Protein **13g** ║ Fat **16g** (Sat Fat 3g, Poly 1g, Mono 10g)
Carbohydrate **23g** ║ Fibre **9g**

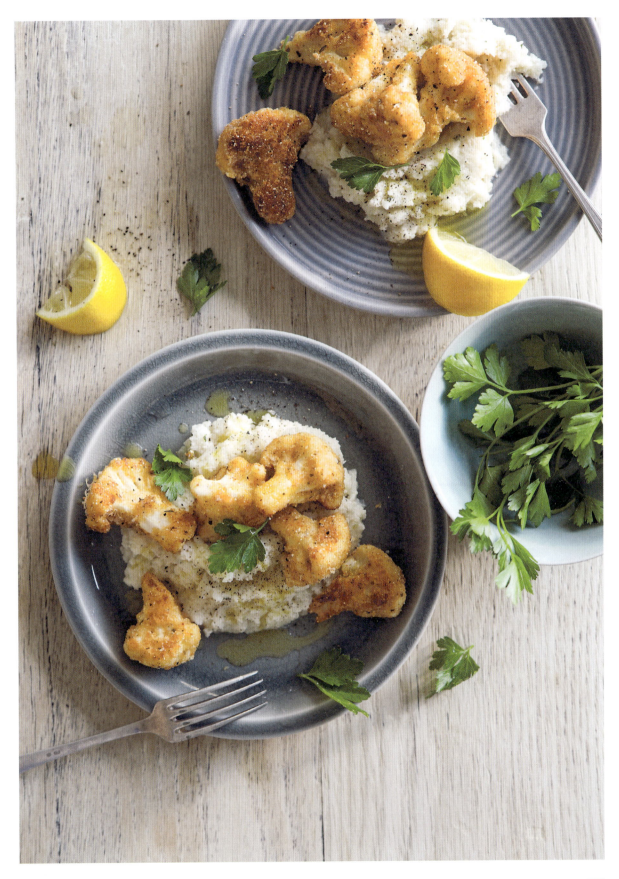

WHAT'S THE BIG DEAL WITH SUGAR?

Media headlines over the past few years would have us believe that sugar is to blame for the obesity epidemic and pretty much every health woe. Of course, it is not. There is no one single dietary factor that is to blame for our health statistics – the associations between diet and health are much more complex.

Nevertheless, collectively we are eating too much added sugar and that is contributing to all sorts of health issues, not least dental health.

For the most part, the encouragement away from sugar is a good thing. If your family have ditched completely, or at least cut down on, soft drinks, biscuits and lollies, you've made a very positive move.

The important distinction is between added sugar and naturally present sugars that are intrinsic to whole foods such as fruit, milk and yoghurt. These foods bring with them a wealth of nutrients and phytochemicals, including fibre, vitamins, minerals and antioxidants. Such a complete nutrition package is entirely different to sugar that has been extracted and refined from a plant, removing all other nutrients in the process, and then added to a highly processed food.

The World Health Organization has recommended that we consume less than 12 teaspoons of added sugar a day, with a further recommendation that, primarily for dental health, we should eat less than 6 teaspoons. These recommendations are for added sugars and not those naturally present in foods. However, current food labelling doesn't differentiate between them. The sugar content on the nutrition information panel refers to total sugars.

Knowing the different names that sugar can be listed under means that you won't be fooled by misleading ingredients lists and health claims.

You can only see if sugars have been added by reading the ingredients list and looking for all the different types of sugars that are added to foods. And there are so many names to look for! Plus, often several types of sugars are used. Here are some of the ways that sugar is listed:

→ Sugar
→ Glucose syrup
→ Words ending in '-ose', e.g. sucrose, dextrose, fructose, glucose, maltose, lactose
→ Brown rice syrup
→ Agave syrup or nectar
→ Coconut sugar or nectar
→ Molasses
→ Honey
→ Maple syrup.

The higher up the ingredients list the sugar is found, the higher the sugar content, but if there are also natural sugars in the food, you can't figure out how much of the total is added. A fruit yoghurt is a good example. The total sugars on the nutrition panel includes the natural sugars that are present in the yoghurt and fruit, as well as any sugar added. There is currently a campaign to rectify this on our labelling, so hopefully we will see a change in the future.

The other ingredient to watch out for is maltodextrin. It is increasingly being used in low-sugar products as technically it is refined starch and therefore not included in the grams of sugar on the nutrition panel. However, maltodextrin is highly refined starch, meaning it has been broken down into short chains. We can break these down into the composite glucose units extremely quickly, leading to a sharp rise in blood sugar levels. It has the same kilojoules as sugar, yet a higher GI. Is it healthier to replace sugar with maltodextrin? Not in our book!

Are some sugars healthier?

You'll see in our recipes that we prefer using honey and pure maple syrup (not flavoured maple syrup, as this is glucose syrup with flavourings attempting to replicate the real thing). That's because the 'real' versions of these foods are unrefined sugars. They may even have some health benefits.

Honey, for example, contains prebiotics that have been shown to benefit the gut microbiome. Both honey and maple syrup provide other potentially beneficial compounds such as antioxidants or small levels of nutrients, but to be honest you'll find much higher levels in other foods. The bottom line is that while we favour these as our sweeteners, they are still added sugars and so you need to be mindful of quantities.

Some sugars are promoted as being healthier, including coconut sugar, coconut nectar and brown rice syrup. The latter is even used in so-called 'sugar free' recipes, which is utter nonsense. Brown rice syrup (sometimes called rice malt syrup) is a mixture of glucose, maltose and maltotriose – all sugars. The reason that it's promoted as healthy is that it is fructose free and there are some concerns over high intakes of added fructose. On the flip side, brown rice syrup has an extremely high GI of 98, meaning it will raise blood glucose levels rapidly. Don't be fooled by its false health halo.

Coconut sugar is another example of misleading marketing. It is made from sap from the spikes of coconut palms and is a mixture of sucrose, glucose and fructose... so yes, it is another sugar. Sugars are the form of carbohydrate in many plants, used to fuel their own growth. Why should sugars extracted from one plant over another be any healthier? The true difference is in price – coconut sugar is about 20 times the price of regular white sugar! Don't buy into the nonsense. All added sugars should be limited and the only reason to buy one type of sugar over another is for flavour or a particular culinary application (caramelisation, for example, with brown sugar).

What about artificial and natural sweeteners?

With the attention given to reducing sugar, there has been a rise in the use of alternative sweeteners in food products.

Common artificial sweeteners include aspartame (E951), acesulphame potassium (E950), cyclamate (E952) and sucralose (E955). You'll find these in no-sugar and diet versions of soft drinks, yoghurts, sweetener tablets, protein powders and bars, chewing gum and mints, jellies and cordials.

There has been much scaremongering on the internet over whether these are safe to consume. The reality is that many of the claims made have been disproven with pretty rigorous research. Nevertheless, we don't recommend these as a regular addition in your family's diet. They have been shown to have a detrimental effect on the gut microbiome and this may have a whole variety of negative knock-on effects that impact weight, appetite and glucose control.

The concerns over these artificial additives has led to increased use of so-called 'natural' sweeteners. Stevia is the most common, but you might also come across monk fruit. These are not really as natural as claimed. The sweet compounds are extracted from the plant and highly refined. In the case of stevia, these compounds are called steviol glycosides and they are incredibly sweet. To turn stevia into a granular white product that can be used like sugar, it is mixed in minute quantities with erythritol. Read the ingredients list of a stevia sweetener and you'll see that in almost every case, erythritol makes up some 99% of the product.

Erythritol (E968) is what is called a nutritive sweetener. This category also includes xylitol (E967), sorbitol (E420) and mannitol (E421). They do provide some kilojoules, but much less than sugar. They are very badly digested and therefore have a minimal impact on blood glucose levels. The other plus is that the oral bacteria can't break them down and so they are tooth-friendly. However, they can result in excessive flatulence and diarrhoea when over-consumed and some people are more susceptible than others. Erythritol tends to be better tolerated since most of it is absorbed and then excreted unchanged in urine.

Small amounts of any of the above are generally not a problem and if they help you to move away from too much added sugar, then terrific. However, the significant problem with all of them is that they continue to encourage a preference for sweet foods. Most research doesn't show that they benefit weight control, which may be because they don't really have the same satiating taste – it seems we can't fool the brain into tasting sweetness without having the associated kilojoules.

Take-home messages

Sugar is not toxic – glucose is sugar, after all, and it runs in our bloodstream to fuel cells all over the body. However, eating too many foods with high levels of added sugars means you are consuming lots of kilojoules without many nutrients alongside. Focus on limiting your added sugars and instead get your sweet fix from natural foods as much as possible, such as fruit and natural yoghurt.

A little honey or pure maple syrup are our favoured sweeteners, but they are still sugars, so be sure to use them sparingly.

Alternative sweeteners, whether natural or artificial, are not a panacea to having sweet foods. A 'no added sugar' label tends to make a product appear healthy, but is it really? A biscuit that's made from white flour, butter and a sweetener is still not healthy, particularly if the sugar-free label gives you an unlimited licence to eat them and you eat the whole packet instead of two of the real thing!

Whether considered artificial or natural, sweeteners are not necessarily any healthier than simply using a little sugar.

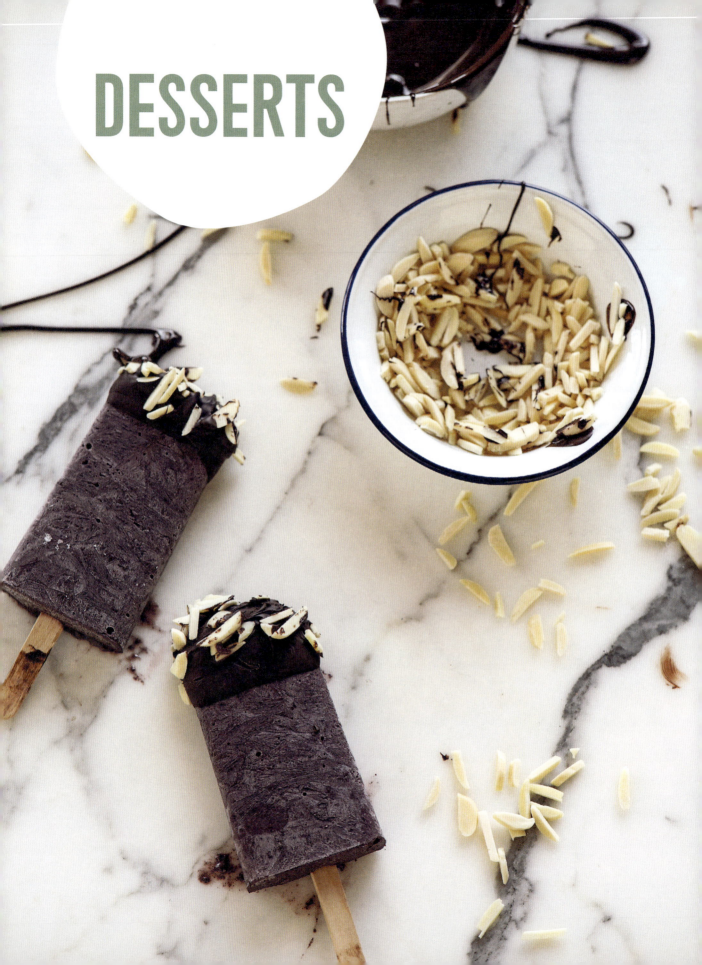

DESSERTS

BANANA ACAI CHOC POPSICLES

PREP TIME: 15 MINUTES, PLUS FREEZING **COOK TIME: 5 MINUTES**

Homemade popsicles are a great way to use up ripe bananas. When they're turning brown in the fruit bowl, peel and freeze them to use in this recipe. Substitute any other frozen fruit you like such as berries, mango or kiwifruit.

SERVES 6

2 bananas, chopped
2 x 100 g acai sachets
⅓ cup (80 ml) coconut milk
1 tablespoon slivered almonds
120 g dark chocolate (70% cocoa),
   finely chopped

Blend the bananas, acai and coconut milk in a blender until smooth. Insert ice-cream sticks into six small popsicle moulds. Pour in the banana mixture and freeze for at least 2–3 hours or until firm.

Toast the almonds in a dry frying pan over low heat until slightly golden. Transfer to a bowl and set aside to cool.

Put the chocolate in a microwave-safe bowl and heat on Medium in 20-second bursts, stirring after each time, until the chocolate is melted and smooth. Alternatively, put the chocolate in a heatproof bowl and set it over a saucepan of simmering water, making sure the water doesn't touch the bowl. Stir until the chocolate is melted and smooth. Allow the chocolate to cool slightly.

Line an airtight container with baking paper.

Remove the popsicles from the moulds. Working with one at a time, carefully dip the end of each popsicle into the melted chocolate and then into the almonds. Place in the container. Return to the freezer for 30 minutes before serving, or store in the freezer for up to a month.

TIP

→ You might want to melt a little more chocolate than you need to make it easier to dip the popsicles.

nutrition per popsicle Energy **820kJ** ‖ Protein **4g** ‖ Fat **12g** (Sat Fat 7g, Poly <1g, Mono 4g)
Carbohydrate **17g** ‖ Fibre **2g**

BLACK RICE PUDDING

PREP TIME: **10 MINUTES**   COOK TIME: **55 MINUTES**

This is a great pudding to make for the kids using left-over cooked black rice. Use whatever milk you have in the fridge. Full-fat milk will increase the kilojoules, of course, but it will also make a richer, creamier pudding.

SERVES 4

1 cup (250 ml) milk
100 ml coconut milk
1 teaspoon vanilla bean paste
2 tablespoons honey
2 large eggs
1 cup (140 g) cooked black rice
¼ teaspoon ground cinnamon

Put the milk, coconut milk, vanilla bean paste and honey in a saucepan. Bring to a simmer over medium heat, stirring to combine.

Whisk the eggs in a bowl.

Carefully add a ladleful of the hot coconut milk mixture to the eggs, whisking constantly. Using a sieve, strain the egg mixture back into the saucepan to ensure it is completely smooth. Stir to combine.

Reduce the heat to medium–low. Cook, stirring, for about 5–8 minutes or until the mixture thickens enough to coat the back of a wooden spoon.

Spread the cooked black rice over the base of a 20 cm square ovenproof dish. Pour in the coconut milk mixture and sprinkle the cinnamon over the top.

Bake for 40 minutes or until the custard is set.

nutrition per serve   Energy **780kJ** ‖ Protein **8g** ‖ Fat **7g** (Sat Fat 5g, Poly <1g, Mono 1g)
Carbohydrate **23g** ‖ Fibre **1g**

FRUIT SALAD WITH HAZELNUTS, LIME AND CHOCOLATE SHAVINGS

PREP TIME: 15 MINUTES 👜 **COOK TIME: NIL**

It's hard to beat a simple fruit salad for a light, nutritious but deliciously tasty dessert. Take advantage of the enormous variety of seasonal fruit on offer and experiment with different combinations. Dress it up with the grated zest of a lime, orange or lemon, add some chopped nuts or toasted coconut, or grate a little dark chocolate over the top.

SERVES 4

- 200 g papaya, skin and seeds removed, diced
- 1 cup (170 g) diced rockmelon
- 120 g blueberries
- 120 g blackberries
- 1 handful mint leaves
- Juice of 1 lime
- 1 cup (260 g) Greek-style yoghurt
- ¼ cup (30 g) hazelnuts, roughly chopped
- 20 g dark chocolate

Combine the papaya, rockmelon and berries in a large bowl. Sprinkle with the mint and lime juice and gently toss together.

Divide the fruit salad among four bowls. Add a big spoonful of yoghurt to each serve, sprinkle with the nuts and grate or shave the chocolate over the top.

TIPS

→ Make a big container of fruit salad, using any fruit in season. Keep in the fridge for up to 5 days to use on breakfast cereal, muesli or porridge, for snacks and desserts.

→ Try other toppings, such as coconut, grated citrus zest, chopped almonds or macadamia nuts, chia seeds, pepitas (pumpkin seeds), poppy seeds or sunflower seeds.

→ This is a fabulous dessert for entertaining. Serve the fruit on a large board or platter, topped with the nuts, mint, chocolate and some grated lime zest.

nutrition per serve | Energy **800kJ** | Protein **8g** | Fat **8g** (Sat Fat 2g, Poly <1g, Mono 5g)
Carbohydrate **19g** | Fibre **6g**

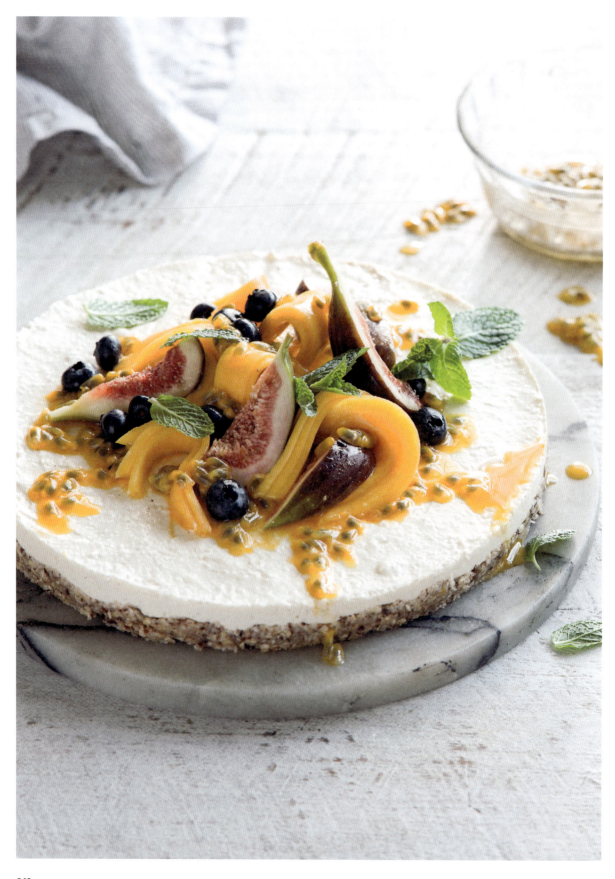

YOGHURT LABNEH CHEESECAKE

PREP TIME: 15 MINUTES, PLUS 2½ HOURS CHILLING **COOK TIME: NIL**

Decorate the cheesecake with seasonal fruit, such as passionfruit pulp, sliced mango, blueberries, raspberries, strawberries, sliced figs or citrus segments.

SERVES 12

BASE
1 cup (120 g) raw hazelnuts
⅔ cup (70 g) rolled oats
⅓ cup (30 g) shredded coconut
25 g sunflower seeds
Grated zest of 1 lemon
1½ tablespoons lemon juice
2 tablespoons tahini
60 g honey

FILLING
10 g sachet gelatine
2 tablespoons boiling water
250 g light cream cheese, softened
250 g labneh (page 48 or
    store-bought)
2 tablespoons pure maple syrup
1 teaspoon vanilla bean paste

TOPPING
Seasonal fresh fruit
Mint leaves

Line the base of a 22 cm round spring-form cake tin with baking paper.

To make the base, chop the hazelnuts, rolled oats, coconut, sunflower seeds and lemon zest in a food processor until the mixture resembles coarse sand. With the motor running, slowly pour in the lemon juice, tahini and honey and process until the mixture comes together.

Tip the nut mixture into the lined tin and press the mixture evenly over the base. Chill for 30 minutes.

To make the filling, combine the gelatine and boiling water in a small bowl. Stir until the gelatine has dissolved.

Combine the softened cream cheese, labneh, maple syrup and vanilla bean paste in the cleaned food processor bowl. Process until combined.

Strain the gelatine to ensure there are no lumps, then add it to the cream cheese mixture and process until smooth.

Pour the filling over the base and smooth the surface. Gently tap the tin on the bench to release any air pockets. Place in the fridge to set for 2 hours or overnight.

Just before serving, carefully release the cheesecake from the tin and transfer it to a plate. Decorate the top with the fruit and mint leaves.

nutrition per serve   Energy **1000kJ** ‖ Protein **7g** ‖ Fat **18g** (Sat Fat 7g, Poly 2g, Mono 8g)
Carbohydrate **12g** ‖ Fibre **3g**
(without topping)

STRAWBERRY SHORTCAKE

PREP TIME: **15 MINUTES, PLUS 10 MINUTES SOAKING** COOK TIME: **30 MINUTES**

This is a delicious dessert to make for a weekend treat. Serve it with a dollop of Greek-style yoghurt or with vanilla ice cream. You can top it with any fruit you like in place of the strawberries.

SERVES 6–8

8 pitted medjool dates
135 g wholemeal plain flour
½ cup (50 g) almond meal
3 teaspoons cocoa powder
1 teaspoon baking powder
Pinch of salt
1 teaspoon vanilla bean paste
½ cup (125 ml) mild-flavoured
   extra virgin olive oil
Juice of 1 orange
1 tablespoon pure maple syrup
¼ teaspoon balsamic vinegar
250 g strawberries, sliced
Grated dark chocolate, to garnish

Soak the dates in boiling water for 10 minutes, then drain.

Preheat the oven to 160°C. Line the base of a 22 cm round spring-form cake tin with baking paper.

Blend the flour, almond meal, cocoa powder, baking powder and salt in a food processor until combined. With the motor running, add the vanilla bean paste and then the dates, one at a time. Slowly pour in the oil and process until combined. Tip the mixture into the lined tin and press it evenly over the base and a third of the way up the side.

Bake the tart shell for 20 minutes. Remove from the oven and set aside to cool in the tin.

Combine the orange juice, maple syrup and vinegar in a small saucepan and cook over medium–low heat until reduced by half. Strain through a sieve.

Arrange the sliced strawberries in the shell and brush them with the glaze. Sprinkle the chocolate over the strawberries.

TIP

→ For an adults-only version, soak the strawberries in ¼ cup (60 ml) Cointreau before pouring them into the tart shell.

nutrition per serve (8 serves)   Energy **1140kJ** ‖ Protein **4g** ‖ Fat **19g** (Sat Fat 3g, Poly 2g, Mono 13g)
Carbohydrate **20g** ‖ Fibre **5g**

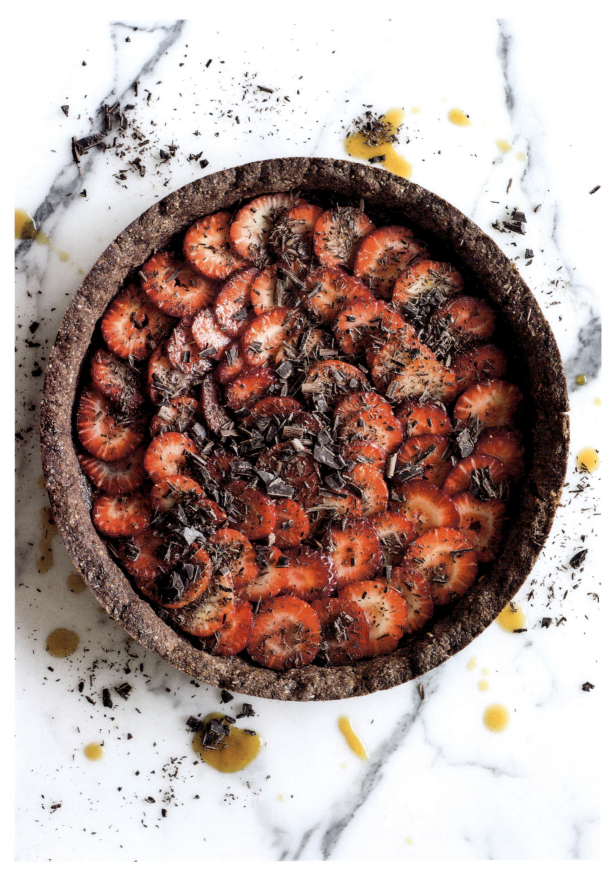

DARK CHOC 'BERRY RIPE'

PREP TIME: **15 MINUTES + FREEZING** COOK TIME: **5 MINUTES**

These little treats are for those moments when you need something sweet.
Keep them in the fridge, or freeze them for an ice-cold treat.

MAKES 26

2 cups (250 g) frozen mixed berries
6 pitted medjool dates
1 cup (90 g) desiccated coconut
200 g dark couverture chocolate
   (minimum 53% cocoa solids),
   finely chopped

Put the berries in a food processor and blitz until combined. Add the dates, one at a time, and blitz until smooth after each addition. Stir in the coconut.

Spoon the berry mixture into ice-cube trays, pressing firmly and levelling the top. Freeze for at least 1 hour or until firm.

Put the chocolate in a microwave-safe bowl and heat on Low in 20-second bursts, stirring after each time, until the chocolate is melted and smooth. Alternatively, put the chocolate in a heatproof bowl and set it over a saucepan of simmering water, making sure the water doesn't touch the bowl. Stir until the chocolate is melted and smooth. Allow the chocolate to cool slightly.

Line an airtight container with baking paper.

Carefully pop the berry cubes out of the ice-cube trays. Using two forks, dip one cube at a time into the melted chocolate. Allow the chocolate to drain over the bowl for a few seconds before transferring the chocolate-coated berry cube to the lined container. When all of the berry cubes have been coated with chocolate, put the lid on the container and transfer to the fridge to set.

Store in the fridge for 10 days or freeze for up to 2 months.

nutrition per serve   Energy **520kJ** ‖ Protein **1g** ‖ Fat **9g** (Sat Fat 7g, Poly 0g, Mono <2g)
Carbohydrate **9g** ‖ Fibre **2g**

NUTTY CHOC BANANA 'ICE CREAM'

PREP TIME: **5 MINUTES** COOK TIME: **NIL**

This recipe couldn't be simpler and it honestly tastes divine, perfect for a healthier ice-creamy treat. Substitute any nut butter you like.

SERVES 4 (MAKES 8 POPSICLES)

4 bananas, frozen (about 340 g in total)
120 g cashew nut butter
2 tablespoons cocoa powder
150 ml coconut water

Combine the frozen bananas, nut butter, cocoa and coconut water in a blender. Blend until smooth.

Serve the 'ice cream' immediately in bowls, or pour it into eight popsicle moulds and freeze until very firm.

TIP

→ You can use whatever nut butter you like in this recipe.

nutrition per serve (4 serves) Energy **1160kJ** ‖ Protein **7g** ‖ Fat **15g** (Sat Fat 3g, Poly 2g, Mono 9g)
Carbohydrate **26g** ‖ Fibre **5g**

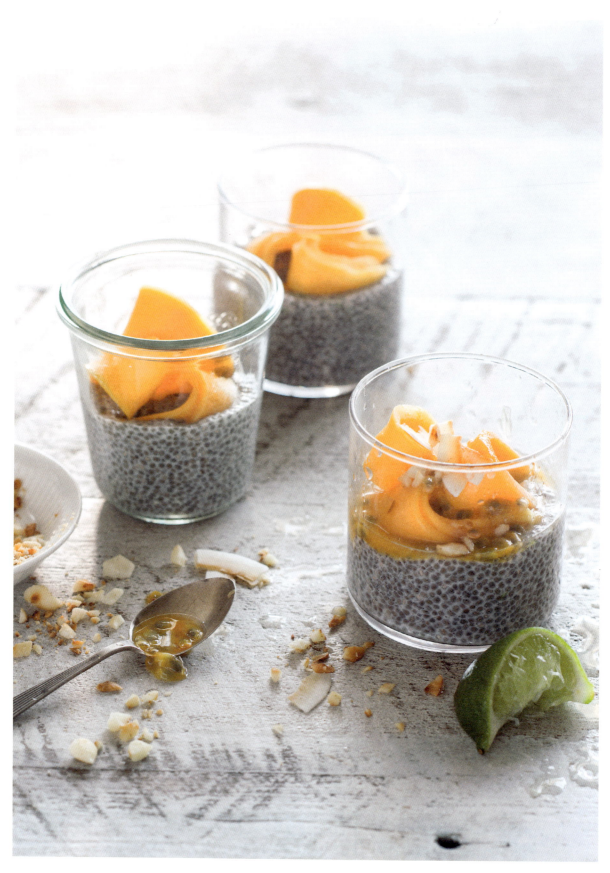

CHIA PUDDINGS WITH MANGO, LIME AND MACADAMIA

PREP TIME: 15 MINUTES, PLUS 2 HOURS SETTING COOK TIME: **5 MINUTES**

This is a gorgeous summer dessert, deliciously light and fresh. Chia seeds are rich in plant omega-3 fats, antioxidants, nutrients and fibre. The soluble fibre is on the outside of the seeds and this is what absorbs water, swelling to create a gel that forms the basis for this pudding.

SERVES 4

60 g chia seeds
300 ml milk
1 teaspoon vanilla bean paste
¼ cup (30 g) macadamia nuts, roughly chopped
1 tablespoon shredded or flaked coconut
Grated zest of 1 lime
Juice of ½ lime
1 large mango cheek, sliced into thin ribbons
Pulp of 2 passionfruit
Lime wedges, to serve

Whisk the chia seeds, milk and vanilla bean paste in a glass container with a lid. Place in the fridge to set for at least 2 hours.

Toast the macadamias in a small frying pan over medium–low heat for 1–2 minutes or until slightly golden. Remove from the pan and set aside.

Lightly toast the coconut in the same pan until just golden. Remove from the pan immediately as the coconut will continue to brown. Set aside to cool.

Once the chia pudding has thickened, add the lime zest and lime juice. Gently stir to combine.

Divide the chia pudding among four serving bowls or glasses. Top with the mango ribbons and passionfruit, then sprinkle with the toasted macadamias and coconut. Serve with lime wedges for an extra squeeze of juice.

TIPS

→ The pudding base can be stored in the fridge for up to 5 days.
→ Serve the puddings with any seasonal fruit – kiwifruit, berries, orange, blood orange, guava, stone fruit, banana or figs.

nutrition per serve   Energy **570kJ** ‖ Protein **5g** ‖ Fat **9g** (Sat Fat 2g, Poly 3g, Mono 4g)
Carbohydrate **7g** ‖ Fibre **6g**

MAPLE-BAKED BANANA WITH HOMEMADE CUSTARD

PREP TIME: 5 MINUTES **COOK TIME: 25 MINUTES**

There's nothing wrong with having custard powder in the pantry to make a quick dessert, but there's no doubt that fresh custard like this is infinitely tastier. Ready-made custard tends to be extremely sweet, whereas making it yourself allows you to control the amount of added sugar.

SERVES 4

4 bananas
2 teaspoons pure maple syrup
½ teaspoon freshly grated nutmeg

CUSTARD
1 cup (250 ml) milk
1 teaspoon vanilla bean paste
¼ teaspoon ground cinnamon
4 egg yolks
1 tablespoon honey
2 teaspoons arrowroot

Preheat the oven to 180°C.

Cut the bananas in half lengthways, keeping the skin on. Brush with the maple syrup and sprinkle with the nutmeg. Place the bananas on a baking tray and bake for 25 minutes or until soft.

Meanwhile, to make the custard, heat the milk, vanilla bean paste and cinnamon in a small saucepan over medium heat until almost boiling. Remove from the heat.

Whisk the egg yolks, honey and arrowroot in a heatproof bowl until well combined.

Slowly pour the hot milk into the egg mixture while whisking. Pour the mixture back into the saucepan and stir over low heat until the custard has thickened and coats the back of a wooden spoon.

Serve the baked bananas with the warm custard.

TIPS

→ Flavour the custard with grated orange, lemon or lime zest.
→ Before baking the bananas, sprinkle them with a little coconut or chopped nuts.

nutrition per serve   Energy **880kJ** ‖ Protein **6g** ‖ Fat **6g** (Sat Fat 2g, Poly <1g, Mono 2g)
Carbohydrate **32g** ‖ Fibre **3g**

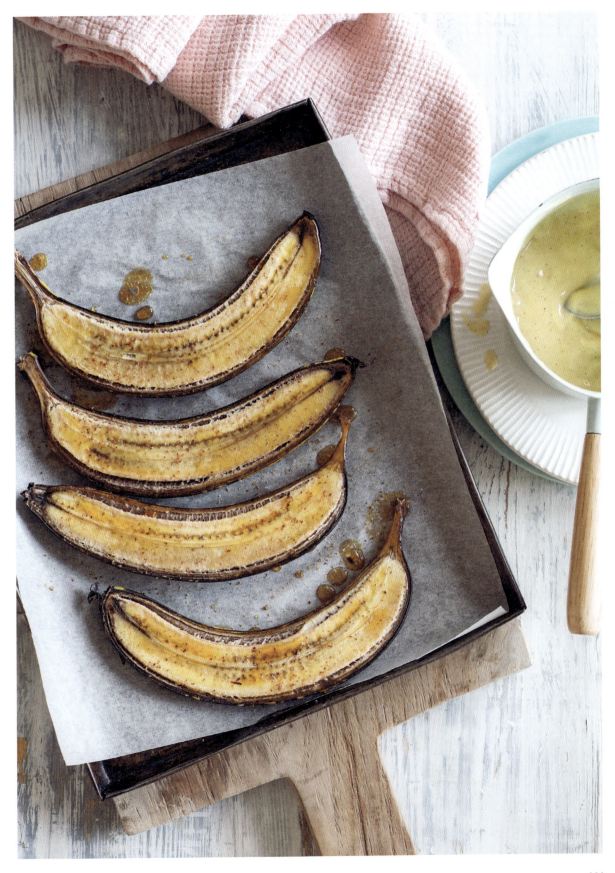

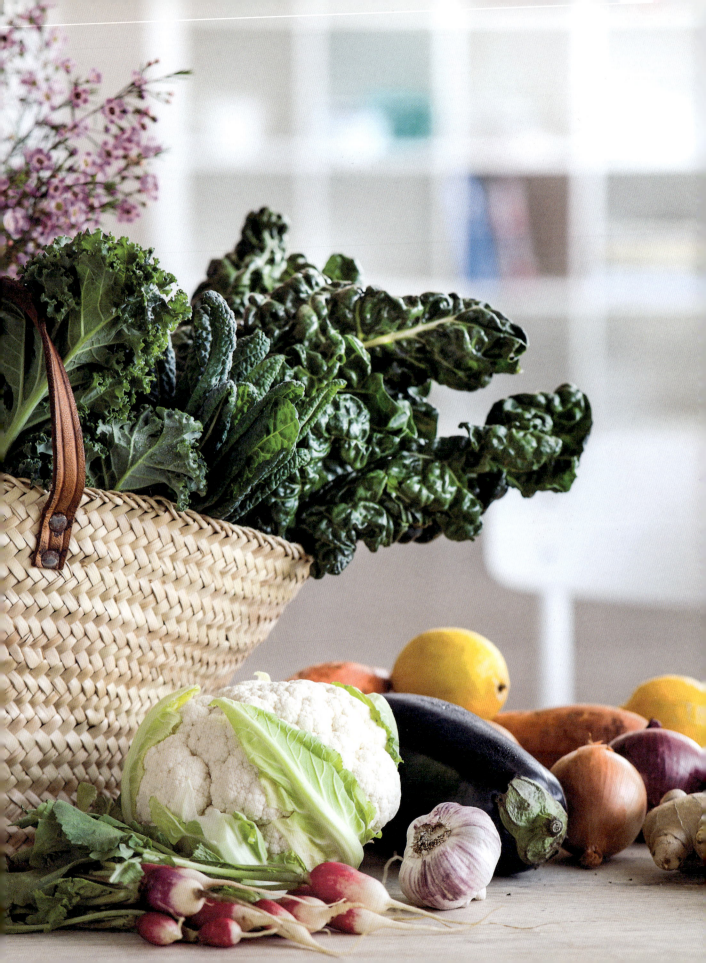

PANTRY ESSENTIALS

When your pantry is stocked with the essentials, you're always ready to whip up a quick, healthy meal, even if the fridge is practically empty. Keeping your pantry well organised will also make life easier. Do a regular audit – empty everything onto the kitchen bench and get rid of anything that's out of date. Wipe out all the shelves and then reorganise your pantry, using tubs, baskets or tiered shelf inserts to make it easier to find all your ingredients. Store the items that you use most often at eye level and within easy reach. Put any items that you don't want to be tempted by up high and out of sight. That way, your willpower isn't tested every time you open the pantry. Removing temptation will make healthy eating the easiest and most effortless choice for everyone.

We've listed the items that we frequently use in our cooking. Use this list as a guide and build your own essential pantry that's based on your family's preferences.

Oils, vinegars and sauces

EXTRA VIRGIN OLIVE OIL

This is really the only oil you need. And the fresher it is, the better. Always buy extra virgin olive oil, as oils labelled simply as 'olive oil' have been refined and they lack many of the wonderful protective polyphenols and other protective compounds that are found in true extra virgin olive oil. It is a myth that you cannot cook with extra virgin olive oil. Research has clearly shown that not only is it safe to cook with, it is the safest of the common supermarket oils. While some oils, including canola and sunflower oils, break down during cooking, producing potentially harmful chemicals, extra virgin olive oil is remarkably resilient. The other amazing thing about extra virgin olive oil is that it improves the absorption and availability of many of the protective plant compounds, such as antioxidants, that are found in vegies. Use it to roast or stir-fry, barbecue, drizzle over steamed or microwaved vegies and as the base for your salad dressings. You can even use it in baking.

ALTERNATIVE OILS

These optional, healthy choices can be terrific for flavour in a dressing or other dish: avocado oil, cold-pressed nut oils, flaxseed oil (keep this in the fridge once opened and never cook with it, as it is a fragile oil) and sesame oil (a must for flavouring some Asian dishes, but don't heat this oil – add it at the end of cooking).

VINEGAR

It's a good idea to have a selection of different vinegars, but you certainly don't need them all. White vinegar is added to the cooking water when poaching eggs and pickling vegetables. Balsamic, red wine, white wine and sherry vinegars are all terrific for salad dressings, marinades and sauces. Rice vinegar is often used in Asian cooking. You can keep vinegars pretty much indefinitely, so you can have a few varieties in the pantry without concerns of adding to food waste, although they may lose some flavour after a few years.

SOY SAUCE OR TAMARI

Tamari is a Japanese-style soy sauce. It is gluten free, but you will also find gluten-free soy sauces on the market. These are very salty sauces, so use them sparingly and don't use additional salt. You can also purchase salt-reduced varieties.

OTHER ASIAN SAUCES

Oyster sauce and fish sauce are also very salty, so use them sparingly. Sweet chilli sauce is extremely high in added sugar, so limit how much you use. Mirin is a subtly flavoured rice wine that's used in Japanese cooking. It's gorgeous in homemade teriyaki-style marinades for meat, fish or tofu. Use it to make your own hoisin sauce (page 105). It's so much better than bought hoisin, but you can purchase it if you prefer.

POMEGRANATE MOLASSES

This is essentially pomegranate juice, reduced to a thick, slightly sticky, tart concentrate. An essential ingredient in many Middle Eastern dishes, it's lovely in dressings and marinades.

HOT CHILLI SAUCE

Hot chilli sauce is great for adding a little fire to your stir-fries, marinades, sauces or finished dishes for those who like it hot. Take your pick from sriracha, sambal oelek, chipotle, Tabasco and a whole lot more.

Bottles, tins and jars

PASSATA

Passata is simply puréed tomatoes, sometimes with added herbs. It's brilliant for making sauces without 'bits' for fussy eaters! Look for varieties that don't contain added salt so that you can control how much salt you add to your meals (if any).

TOMATOES

Tinned tomatoes are perfect for quick and easy sauces, soups and casseroles. Look for those without added salt or other additives – read the ingredients list and choose one that contains only tomatoes and tomato juice.

CORN KERNELS

Corn is a rich source of fibre and a good source of B-group vitamins that are needed to turn our food into energy in the body. Tinned corn kernels are ready to eat and great for adding to salads, sandwich fillings, pasta dishes and rice dishes.

BEETROOT

Not many vegies are suitable for canning as they lose their texture and often nutrients as well. Beetroot is one of the few exceptions. It's great for popping in homemade burgers, sandwiches and wraps.

FISH

Tinned tuna, salmon, mackerel and sardines all make it easy to eat more oily fish, which contains the anti-inflammatory omega-3 fats. Look for those bearing a sustainable seafood logo.

CAPERS

You'll find these pickled, edible flower buds packed in salt or a liquid brine in jars. They add a wonderful burst of flavour to Mediterranean-style dishes. Be sure to rinse them first to get rid of the excess salt.

OLIVES

Olives are another key ingredient in Mediterranean cooking. They're exceptionally high in beneficial polyphenols. However, they are very high in salt as they are pickled in brine. Avoid adding extra salt to dishes where olives feature prominently.

SOUP

There's nothing wrong with having a few ready-to-eat soups in the pantry in tins, cartons or tetra packs for those times when you want an instant meal or snack. Vegetable and legume-based soups can be a great means of boosting your family's plant food intake. Microwavable packs are convenient for heating at work for lunch, or heating at home to pop into a thermos container for school lunches. Check the ingredients list for any unwanted additives (for more information on reading food labels, see pages 178–179).

Grains

There is a massive difference between refined and wholegrain foods and products. From a health and nutrition view, always seek out the wholegrain option. Wholegrains are associated with less chronic disease and better weight control. The fibre that they contain plays an especially important role in the health of the gut and microbiome, and wholegrain products deliver more nutrients overall.

In today's world we have to think not just about which foods are best for our health, but also which are best for the health of our planet. Fortunately, the two are very closely aligned. The shift towards plant-rich eating, whether or not you also eat animal foods, is key and wholegrains are a wonderfully nutritious, not to mention budget-friendly, addition to your pantry.

Wholegrains tend to have lower GI values, meaning they have less impact on blood glucose levels. They also provide plant protein, something often forgotten as they get labelled as 'carbs'.

The key difference to refined grains is that they contain the outer layers of the grain, meaning you get all the fibre and the many nutrients found there, including B group vitamins and minerals. Wholegrains are also fabulously rich in phytochemicals with antioxidant, anti-inflammatory and other protective qualities.

OATS

Oats stand out amongst grains for their health benefits. Famous for their cholesterol-lowering effect, they are also rich in a diversity of fibre types, including those that fuel healthy gut bugs. Rolled oats are probably the most versatile, but you can also try using steel-cut oats in cooking. Rolled oats can be eaten raw in smoothies or muesli, cooked into muffins or fruit breads, added to pancake mixes, made into porridge or blended to use as a flour.

BARLEY

One of the oldest cultivated grains, barley is worthy of a place in your pantry. It takes some time to cook, which is probably why it tends not to be used as often as oats, but it's not difficult to use. Barley has four times the fibre of brown rice and, like oats, has the types of fermentable fibres that fuel a healthy, diverse microbiome and help to control both cholesterol and blood glucose levels. You can use barley to make a wonderfully nutty, filling, risotto-style dish, add it to soups and winter casseroles, or cook and cool it to toss through salads.

QUINOA

An ancient staple of the Andean region of South America, quinoa was once a trendy 'superfood' of the West. However, quinoa is now more or less mainstream. Admittedly, it is much more expensive than pasta or rice, so won't be suited to all family budgets. Don't feel you have to buy it – no food is an essential for a healthy diet! It's a good option, nevertheless, boasting much higher protein and fibre levels than rice and a good array of vitamins and minerals. Quinoa is also a good option for those who need to follow a gluten-free diet. It's good hot or cold and can be used as a porridge, in salads (it's wonderful in buddha-style bowls), as an alternative to rice with cooked dishes and even in baking as quinoa flour.

RICE

Look for wholegrain varieties of rice. White rice has been polished to remove the outer layers and this results in a huge loss of nutrients, phytochemicals and fibre. Look out for brown basmati rice (basmati has a lower GI than most rice varieties), wild rice (great mixed with other wholegrain rice varieties or with other grains or legumes) and, our favourite, black rice. The wonderful black-purple colour of black rice is thanks to the polyphenols present, making this an especially nutritious grain. All rice varieties are gluten free and are amongst the least allergenic foods, making rice an especially good food for those with food allergies and intolerances.

POLENTA

Polenta is a good gluten-free grain for those who need to follow a gluten-free diet as it is made from whole corn. Its wonderful yellow colour is thanks to the carotenoids present, which are fabulously good for eye health. It's traditionally used in Italian cuisine and served either as a kind of mash (see page 110) or as polenta chips.

OTHER WHOLEGRAINS

Other wholegrains we sometimes use and that are worth experimenting with include bulgur wheat (used to make tabouli); farro (the Italian name for an ancient wheat variety called emmer, farro is fabulous in salads, soups and as a healthier risotto-style dish); freekeh (an ancient Eastern Mediterranean cracked grain made from young, green wheat); teff (a tiny gluten-free grain from

Ethiopia – the flour is terrific for making pancakes and in baking); millet (a small, gluten-free grain that's a great alternative to couscous); buckwheat (called a pseudo-grain as it is actually a seed, but 'acts' more like a grain; it is also gluten free); and wholemeal couscous (made from the same durum wheat flour used in pasta production).

Pasta and noodles

PASTA

The 'carbophobic' era gave pasta an unfairly bad name. Pasta has been a family staple in Italy for many centuries and the idea is likely to have come from Chinese noodles. In fact, although we think of pasta as being Italian, many countries around the world have their own version. Since it's such an ancient food, we can hardly blame pasta for the world getting fatter in the last 50 or so years!

Be reassured that pasta can remain (or be brought back) as a family favourite. It's a budget-friendly food that, when teamed up with other foods, can make a nutritious, tasty meal. It comes down to portion size and the balance with the other ingredients – use the Plate template on page 8 to create your meal.

If you have ever travelled to Italy, you'll have seen that they have a small serve of pasta as a first course and follow it up with meat or fish and lots of vegies. So, for example, instead of having a huge bowl of spaghetti with a mound of bolognese sauce (as is typical in Australia), reduce the serve of pasta, grate or finely dice vegies into the bolognese sauce and perhaps add some tinned beans to stretch the meat further and boost the plant food content, and serve with a lovely green salad dressed with an extra virgin olive oil vinaigrette.

All durum wheat pasta varieties are low GI, helping with blood glucose control, but for full nutritional benefits, opt for wholegrain pasta where possible. If your family really can't get used to the nuttier taste, look for regular pasta that is high in fibre. There are also a range of legume pastas on the market that are made with beans, lentils or chickpeas. Nutritionally these are terrific, but they do taste different. Give them a shot and see if your family like them.

Gluten-free pastas are usually made from corn, potato or rice flour. They tend to have a high GI and so we don't recommend them unless your family truly needs to be eat gluten free. Even then, there are healthier gluten-free wholegrain food options.

NOODLES

It can be harder to find wholegrain noodles, but they are starting to appear as the interest in plant-rich eating grows. One of our favourites are traditional Japanese soba noodles. Look for those that are 100% buckwheat. These are also gluten free for those that require it. Some brands use a mixture of refined wheat flour and buckwheat so they are not entirely wholegrain, nor gluten free.

You're probably already aware that '2 minute' and 'pot' noodles are not the best. Sometimes the noodles are deep-fried before being dried and these can be significant sources of trans fats, the worst for health. The flavour sachets are full of artificial additives and tend to be extremely high in salt. There are better versions available that are not fried and are additive-free, but they are still a low-nutrient food and should therefore not be an everyday food for kids. Make your own quick noodle dishes instead with vegies and a protein-rich food for balance.

Breads and cereals

BREAD

Almost every country around the world has their own version of bread and humans have been eating it since ancient times. There are, however, big differences in the potential health impact of modern, fast-produced bread made with refined white flour – the average supermarket white sliced loaf – or those made with refined white flour and added sugar – burger buns – compared with a traditionally produced sourdough loaf made with 100% wholegrain flour.

The fermentation process used to produce sourdough bread lowers the GI, so it may have less impact on your blood glucose levels. It does make a chewier bread that may not be to the whole family's taste or be easy for the kids to eat as a lunchbox sandwich.

The most important thing is to choose a wholegrain bread. These breads are made with flour milled from intact grains so that you benefit from all the fibre, nutrients and phytochemicals found in the outer layers of the grain.

Look for bread with different types of grains, including ancient varieties of common grains. For example, spelt, emmer and einkorn are all ancient wheat varieties. While it really isn't known if these are any healthier, some people who experience digestive issues after eating bread made with modern wheat report no such issues with bread made from such ancient grains. In the interests of diversity in our diets, it's a good thing to embrace this variety and ensure we keep a range of plant species alive.

Bread can also be made from all sorts of grains, such as rye, barley and oats, and seeds are often added, including sunflower seeds, poppy seeds, chia seeds, linseeds (another name for flaxseeds) and pepitas (pumpkin seeds), and legumes, such as soy. All of these ingredients are nutritious additions to bread and lend a diversity of fibre types, vitamins, minerals and other beneficial plant compounds.

It's important to note that multigrain bread is not the same as wholegrain bread. Look at the ingredients list on multigrain bread and you will usually see that 'wheat flour' is listed first. This is refined white flour. Some wholegrain flour and/or various cracked grains and seeds are then added, making multigrain a step up from white bread.

If your kids are so accustomed to white bread that you find it hard to get them to switch, at least buy white bread that's labelled as low GI and high fibre. There are several of these on offer in most supermarkets. Next, try a smooth wholemeal bread with no 'bits'. You can even make sandwiches with one slice of wholemeal and one slice of white bread if that helps. As they get used to different types of bread, introduce more varieties and eventually you'll get them used to wholegrain.

FLOUR

If you are not a frequent baker, try to buy your flour in small quantities as the freshness of flour does matter. In warmer climates there is also the problem of little bugs growing in your flour. If you have room, keeping your flour in the freezer will avoid this problem.

Wholegrain or wholemeal flours are the healthiest choices, although admittedly they make denser, heavier baked goods. Try mixing them with legume flours such as besan (chickpea flour) or lupin flour to lighten the end result and boost the nutrition at the same time.

Cornflour is a must for thickening gravies and sauces. Regular white flour is best for making a white sauce or béchamel sauce and the quantity used is small. If you're making a birthday cake or other special occasion treat, use the flour that's recommended in the recipe! This is not an everyday food.

If your cooking needs to be gluten free, experiment with flours made from brown rice, quinoa, teff, amaranth, arrowroot, sorghum or buckwheat. Buckwheat flour is also brilliant for making pancakes.

BREAKFAST CEREALS

Breakfast cereals tend to divide people, with some thinking they are highly processed junk foods and others an easy, budget-friendly and fast route to breakfast for the whole family. The truth is it depends on which ones you pick.

In all fairness, breakfast cereals have come a long way in the last few years. Manufacturers have made significant shifts to use more wholegrains and to greatly reduce the amount of sugar, salt and artificial additives (such as colours) used in their products. This is great for families, as there is no doubt that a bowl of cereal is the easiest breakfast, particularly since even young kids can help themselves. Cereal is also a major supplier of fibre in Australian diets, and those who don't eat cereal tend to have lower fibre intakes.

Essentially, you want to pick a cereal that has the most fibre and the least added sugar and salt, and with no artificial colourings, flavours or preservatives. Look for the word 'wholegrain' on the front of the pack and check the ingredients list to be sure. You're looking for 'whole wheat' rather than 'wheat', 'brown rice' rather than 'rice', or wholegrains such as oats or barley. You'll find more on reading food labels on pages 178–179, but as a rule of thumb for breakfast cereals, look at the 'per 100g' column (as the serve sizes vary). Choose a cereal that contains at least 10g of fibre, less than 15g of sugar (although if it contains dried fruit, this is better than added refined sugars as they are whole foods with the sugar in the matrix of the food – in this case less than 20g of sugar is acceptable) and less than 400mg sodium (salt).

If the kids are used to one of the less than ideal cereals and you're having a battle to get them to switch, try mixing the cereals together for a little while, gradually shifting the proportions in favour of the healthier one. Good nutrition by stealth sometimes works! Or explain to them why the sugary, coloured cereal is not an everyday food, in age-appropriate language, and relegate it to an occasional treat if they must have it.

MUESLI AND GRANOLA

These are generally good, healthy options as they are based on oats and other wholegrains. The same criteria for breakfast cereals applies, but be aware that crunchy muesli varieties and granola sometimes have oil added in order to toast the grains. This is usually a refined oil rather than extra virgin olive oil or any other unrefined oil, hence it's better to choose those without added oil.

Watch for the added sugar as the crunch often comes from toasting in syrup. There are healthier options now available, with low sugar and plenty of fabulous, healthy additions including seeds, nuts and different wholegrains.

Beans and lentils

Collectively called legumes, this group of plant foods are set to be the superfoods of the next few years as more people make the effort to get more of their protein from plant foods than from animal foods. It's not just a good move for the health of our planet – legumes are packed with good nutrition including protein, fibre, slow-release carbohydrates and several vitamins, minerals and protective plant compounds.

Beans are usually popular foods with kids and they're an easy way to boost nutrition and contribute to the daily vegetable target. Plus they are budget friendly, have a long shelf life and are super convenient, especially direct from the tin.

BEANS

Keep a variety of tinned beans in your pantry. They are terrific for adding to soups, stews and casseroles to make the meat go further, blending to make into dips, mashing as an alternative to potatoes or simply adding to your favourite fresh salads.

Black beans are traditional to many South American dishes. That fabulous purple-black colour comes from the polyphenols present, known to be beneficial for human health. They are also one of the best plant sources of iron if you have a vegetarian in the family. Borlotti and cannellini beans are popular in Italian cooking, red kidney beans are a must for chilli con carne, adzuki beans are a little round red bean popular in Japan, as are young green soybeans called edamame. You'll find all of these and several other varieties in the tinned vegetable section of the supermarket.

You can buy your beans dried, but most you have to soak and cook for a relatively long time before eating. If you're motivated to do so, go for it! Otherwise, there's absolutely nothing wrong with using the tinned varieties.

BAKED BEANS

Baked beans are synonymous with childhood and most kids (and many adults!) love them. With the rightful concerns over sugar added to foods, many have become concerned that baked beans are not a healthy choice, but rest assured that the nutritional pluses far outweigh any potential drawbacks. The total sugar value on the side of the pack is not all added sugar – it includes the naturally present sugars in the tomatoes and the beans. Many brands have also reformulated their product to reduce the amount of sugar added. The nutrition from the beans is the key factor and tinned baked beans are such an easy meal or snack. Older kids can also prepare them for themselves. They're a great snack with cheese after school, and are delicious served on wholemeal muffins with a poached egg for breakfast.

CHICKPEAS

Chickpeas are widely used in Middle Eastern, Indian and Mediterranean cuisines. Use them to make your own hummus (very easy and it tastes so good fresh and still warm from the blender), add them to soups, stews and salads, or bake them to make a crunchy, nut-like snack.

Besan (chickpea flour) is also worth experimenting with. Use it to make pancakes for the kids and add it to the flour mix for muffins and fruit loaves. This adds protein and fibre, while lowering the GI.

PEAS

You probably have a packet of green peas in the freezer, but you can also have dried peas in your pantry. Split green and yellow peas are terrific in soups and Indian dhals. You buy them dried and, unlike most beans, you don't need to soak them before use.

LUPIN

Australian sweet lupin is a food you may not be familiar with, but watch out for it in the coming years as its nutritional attributes are being recognised. This type of lupin does not need soaking and cooking, making it highly versatile. Lupin has a distinctly different nutrient profile to other legumes, being low in carbohydrates and much higher in fibre and protein. You can buy it as lupin flour to use in baking, substituting up to 20% of the wheat flour in a recipe to boost the nutrition, or as lupin flakes. You can use these as an alternative to breadcrumbs for schnitzel and fish, to add to smoothies and as an alternative to lupin flour in baking.

LENTILS

You can buy lentils ready to eat in tins or dried in a packet. You don't have to soak lentils – just cook them directly from the packet. Puy lentils, sometimes called French lentils, hold their shape during cooking, making them terrific in salads. Red and yellow lentils become mushy on cooking and are best used in soups, dhals, curries and casseroles. Green lentils fall somewhere in the middle. Pick the lentil to suit your dish!

Nuts and seeds

Nuts and seeds are terrific additions to your family's diet and most of us do not eat enough of them. The rise in allergies amongst children has not helped, which is a shame because nuts and seeds are incredibly nutrient-dense and have much to offer most members of the family. Plus, they're really tasty! While you can't send nuts to school (at least not to primary schools – high schools all seem to vary in their nut policy), they can, and should be, eaten at home by kids with no allergy.

In general, nuts are a good source of plant protein, they're rich in healthy unsaturated fats, and they provide fibre and an impressive array of vitamins, minerals and beneficial phytochemicals.

Nuts and seeds make great snacks – a bowl of mixed nuts, seeds and berries is delicious, and you can add a little dark chocolate when you feel like something more decadent. Use them as a topping on breakfast cereal and porridge. Add them to smoothies when you need breakfast on the run or a more substantial snack. Scatter them over salads for texture and crunch. And bake them into breads, muffins and snack bars.

Different nuts and seeds have slightly varying nutritional profiles, but all are worthy of a place in your pantry and the more different types you include, the better. Choose from almonds, Brazil nuts, cashews, macadamias, pecans, hazelnuts, pistachios, pine nuts and walnuts. Peanuts are actually a legume, but they're nutritionally similar to tree nuts. Terrific seeds to try are white and black sesame seeds, sunflower seeds, pepitas (pumpkin seeds), poppy seeds, linseeds (also called flaxseeds) and chia seeds.

Coconut

Coconut is not really a nut, but a type of fruit called a 'drupe'. Nutritionally it is quite different to tree nuts. It is exceptionally high in saturated fat and that has made it controversial. The types of saturated fat present are different to those found in animal foods and do not seem to have the same effects on health. Nevertheless, coconut lacks the impressive levels of vitamins, minerals and phytochemicals found in other nuts. There's nothing wrong with using a little desiccated or shredded coconut – these are whole foods that do provide some fibre and they are a tasty ingredient in many recipes. Coconut milk and coconut cream are very energy dense so they are not alternatives to dairy milk, but they are essential for many recipes that are traditional to coconut-growing areas. We use them in small amounts for such recipes.

Seasonings

SALT

Many of us eat far too much salt, but most of it comes from processed foods. If you limit such foods in your family's diet, then you don't need to worry too much about using a little in your cooking. The exception is if any member of the family has high blood pressure or has been told to eat a low-salt diet. Be aware that fancy salts such as Himalayan salt are not healthier than regular table salt. In fact, you are best to use an iodised salt as many people are low in iodine. This mineral is essential for thyroid metabolism and healthy brain development. You can buy both iodised salt flakes and table salt – either way, use it sparingly.

HERBS AND SPICES

Herbs and spices are key for turning a meal into something truly delicious. They also pack a tremendous amount of nutrition into a small package – they top the charts for antioxidant power and many have been used medicinally since ancient times. Of course, quantity matters, so using a pinch every now and again won't have much effect. Use them generously and regularly for best results in terms of taste and nutrition.

We love fresh herbs and if you can grow your own herb garden, you'll always have them fresh to hand. Dried herbs are a good, convenient substitute when fresh are not available. They do need to be relatively fresh for the best flavour, so make sure you use them regularly and check the 'best before' dates.

Our favourite herbs are basil, oregano, parsley, rosemary, mint, thyme, chives, coriander, dill, tarragon and Italian blend.

Our favourite spices are black pepper, chilli, turmeric, paprika (smoked and sweet), coriander (seeds and ground), cumin (seeds and ground), cinnamon (sticks and ground), za'atar, sumac and Chinese five spice.

Sweeteners

HONEY

Honey is a truly unrefined sweetener. Look for pure floral honeys for the best quality as some inferior honeys have been adulterated with glucose syrup. Pure honey even contains some prebiotics that benefit the gut microbiome.

MAPLE SYRUP

Maple syrup is the concentrated sap of Canadian maple trees. Be careful not to confuse maple-flavoured syrups with pure maple syrup. These are usually just a processed glucose syrup with added flavourings to mimic the real thing, and are much cheaper as a result.

HELPFUL KITCHEN UTENSILS AND APPLIANCES

There is some obvious equipment that's essential for cooking, but that list is actually rather short. You really don't need every gadget and appliance on the market to be able to whip up healthy meals for your family. The following items can save you time or simply make it easier to get a meal prepared, cooked and onto the table.

Knives and a knife sharpener

You need at least a couple of good, sharp kitchen knives of different sizes. Nothing is more frustrating than working with blunt knives. Learn to use a steel or purchase a good knife sharpener to keep your blades in top shape. Regularly sharpening knives is essential and it's worth having them sharpened by a professional once a year or so.

Mandolin

Sometimes called a V-slicer, a mandolin is a brilliant tool for shaving meats for sandwiches, slicing vegies super-thin or into julienne strips, making crinkle-cut chips and for various other slicing and dicing jobs, with varying thickness.

Salad dressing shaker

You can, of course, make salad dressings in a screw-top jar. However, a good salad shaker has an internal paddle to help disperse thicker ingredients like honey, mustard or pomegranate molasses. Look for one that has measurements on the side and a spout for easy pouring.

Salad spinner

A salad spinner is an inexpensive yet indispensable tool for washing and drying leafy salad greens. It's a great job to give the kids!

Non-stick saucepans and frying pans

Using non-stick pans makes cooking and cleaning up considerably easier. There have been concerns about chemical leaching from non-stick coatings, but modern pans from reputable manufacturers have been shown to be safe. Buying a set with a few different sizes is usually an economical choice and many sets also include a frying pan. A smaller frying pan is also useful for making omelettes and for frying small quantities of food. If you regularly make pancakes or crepes, a pancake pan is also useful. It has very shallow sides, making it easier to spread the batter out and flip your pancakes.

Cast-iron cookware

This type of cookware is brilliant to cook with, particularly for dishes that you want to start on the stovetop, such as casseroles, then transfer to the oven to cook long and slow. A cast-iron chargrill pan cooks a fabulous steak and creates lovely grill marks on vegies, meat or fish. Cast-iron cookware can be expensive, but it lasts a lifetime.

Grain cooker

Although it's certainly not an essential item as you can simply use a pot on the stove, a grain cooker does make it super easy to cook grains perfectly, every time. It will also keep the cooked grains warm until serving time, making it easier to coordinate the timing of your meal. Some grain cookers have a sauté function that allows you to sauté onions, garlic or other vegetables when making pilafs and risotto-style dishes.

Air fryer

This is a magical appliance for families who love their chips but want to eat healthier. You can make your own thick-cut chips or shoestring fries using potatoes or sweet potatoes in their skins (which ensures you get all of the fibre, nutrients and phytochemicals), tossed in extra virgin olive oil and any spices you like. You can also add other vegetables such as red onion, capsicum, parsnip or zucchini.

Jaffle maker

This is basically a toasted sandwich maker, but it seals the edges of the sandwich to make a jaffle, allowing you to incorporate runnier fillings such as baked beans in tomato sauce. Kids usually love jaffles and they aren't as messy to eat as a toasted sandwich, making them handy for when you need to give them a meal or snack on the run. Older kids can make their own – a baked bean and cheese jaffle as an after-school snack is hard to beat. Check out all our jaffle filling ideas on page 42.

Powerful blender

With a good-quality, powerful blender, you can make nut butters, breadcrumbs, dips such as hummus, dressings, sauces, smooth soups and, of course, smoothies. Blenders can be expensive, but you do get what you pay for. The cheaper ones are unable to achieve the same smooth texture and are not as versatile, and they tend to break far more easily. We don't recommend using a juicer as these remove the pulp and, along with it, most of the fibre and several nutrients and phytochemicals. Whole-food smoothies are a nutritionally superior option.

ACKNOWLEDGEMENTS

From Jo

Without the extraordinarily talented team at Murdoch Books, this book would not have been possible. To my publisher, Corinne Roberts – thank you for having the faith in me to produce another book, for all our brain-storming sessions to come up with the right idea and for your expert guidance along the way. To our editors, Jane Price and Justine Harding: thank you for your meticulous eye for detail. To our fabulous creative team, Vivien Valk, Vanessa Austin, Sarah Odgers and photographer Alan Benson – thank you for bringing our book to life so beautifully. And to Carol Warwick and all of the sales and marketing team: thank you for your enthusiasm in getting this book out there.

A huge thank you to my pal and co-author, Mel. This is our baby! I couldn't have done it without you. How lucky I am to get to collaborate with someone who always makes me laugh, never complains at my requests to change ingredients and has the skills to turn my theory into delicious food. Love you, my friend.

To my manager, Simone Landes – I truly appreciate all your support, guidance and organisational skills in keeping me on track. To my husband, Joel: thank you, my love, for your endless support, encouragement and belief in me. Life is so much more fun with you by my side. To my boys, Oliver and Lewis: thank you for putting up with my nutrition lectures at the dinner table and for eating so many test meals!

Finally, a thank you to you, the reader. I hope this book brings joyful healthy eating into your family home.

From Mel

This book has been an ongoing conversation with my gorgeous friend Jo over many kilometres walking together, any number of fitness sessions, many lunch dates and countless phone messages. This book is a dream come true; thank you, Jo. We had a dream to collaborate all those years ago: your encouragement has never wavered; your positive energy has always challenged me to extend outside my comfort zone. Thank you for always trusting and believing in me. I couldn't be more proud of co-authoring this book with you.

To my beautiful girlfriends (you know who you are), who tirelessly tested and tasted many of my recipes. You graciously provided me with valuable feedback, photo results, thumbs up or down. Thank you for all your time, energy and ongoing encouragement.

To Simone Landes, thank you for taking me under your managing wings. Your support and patience throughout this process has been incredible.

To the fabulous Murdoch publishing team – Corinne, Jane, Vivien, Justine, Sarah, Alan, Vanessa and Carol to name a few – this book was made even more special by your excitement at working with us. Thank you for all the hard work, patience and flexibility through this journey.

To the most important men in my life: my boys, Luke and Hudson, and my husband, Brett. Thank you for always supporting my crazy ideas. You have been through the highs and lows of my long career in and passion for food. You have been around the table, trying all my creations. Luke and Hudson, I hope this book will travel with you as you continue to spread your wings in life.

My love for cooking is made all the more special when it is enjoyed with my beautiful family and incredible friends. My heart is full.

INDEX

Published in 2020 by Murdoch Books, an imprint of Allen & Unwin

Murdoch Books Australia
83 Alexander Street, Crows Nest NSW 2065
Phone: +61 (0)2 8425 0100
murdochbooks.com.au
info@murdochbooks.com.au

Murdoch Books UK
Ormond House, 26–27 Boswell Street,
London, WC1N 3JZ
Phone: +44 (0) 20 8785 5995
murdochbooks.co.uk
info@murdochbooks.co.uk

For corporate orders & custom publishing contact our business
development team at salesenquiries@murdochbooks.com.au

Publisher: Corinne Roberts
Editorial Manager: Jane Price
Creative Manager: Vivien Valk
Designer: Sarah Odgers
Editor: Justine Harding
Cover designer: Trisha Garner
Photography: Alan Benson
Styling: Vanessa Austin
Food Preparation for Photography: Sarah Mayoh, Mandy Sinclair, Melissa Hurwitz
Production Director: Lou Playfair

ISBN 978 1 76052 512 5 Australia
ISBN 978 1 91163 249 8 UK

A cataloguing-in-publication entry
is available from the catalogue of
the National Library of Australia at
nla.gov.au

A catalogue record for this book is available from
the British Library

Colour reproduction by Splitting Image Colour
Studio Pty Ltd, Clayton, Victoria

Printed by C & C Offset Printing Co Ltd, China

TABLESPOON MEASURES: We use Australian 20 ml
(4 teaspoon) tablespoon measures. If you are using
a smaller European 15 ml (3 teaspoon) tablespoon,
add an extra teaspoon of the ingredient for each
tablespoon specified.

The nutritional information provided for each recipe
does not include any accompaniments, unless they
are listed in the ingredients. It has been calculated
with reduced-fat milk and reduced-fat yoghurt.
The values are approximations and can be affected
by biological and seasonal variations in food, the
unknown composition of some manufactured foods
and uncertainty in the dietary database.

Front cover shows, clockwise from top right:
Overnight oats page 40, lunchbox with Vegie ricotta
muffin page 78 and Baked muesli bar page 74,
Chicken laksa page 126 and Ways with toast, page 60.

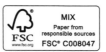